1600+ WODS

by Chris Gale

ISBN - 978-1-71667-474-7

Writer: Chris Gale

Printer: LuLu

Back cover photography: Caitlin Gale

DISCLAIMER

The author and publisher of this material are not responsible in any manner whatsoever for any injury that may occur through following the instructions contained in this material. The activities may be too strenuous or dangerous for some people. The readers should always consult a physician before engaging in them.

About the author

Chris Gale has been the head coach and owner of CrossFit Kenko in Victoria, Australia since 2013. He has overcome brain surgery and found that strength and conditioning, powerlifting. weightlifting, gymnastics and training as a CrossFit athlete has broken all barriers the doctors advised him.

Chris Gale has tried and tested many theories, training protocols and exercise proramming from around the world to compromise his own programming to successfully help his clients achieve their goals.

This book has every workout he has programmed for his Crossfil affiliate since 2013.

For my Family
- Caitlin (wife), Paul (Dad), Sue (Mum), Sarah (sister) also Mojito and Jasper

GLOSSARY

WOD - Workout of the day

AMRAP - As many rounds/reps as possible

KB - Kettlebell

HR push up- Hand release push up

KTE - Knees to elbow

TTB - Toes to bar

KBSHP - Kettlebell sumo high pull

EMOM - Every minute on the minute

OH squat - Overhead squat

C+J - Clean and jerk

AHAP - as heavy as possible

HSPU - Handstand push up

DU - Double under

STO - Shoulder to overhead

GTO - Ground to overhead

MB - Medicine ball

ME - Max effort

PP - push press

PJ - Push jerk

SJ - Split jerk

RFT - Rounds for time

C2B - Chest to bar pull up

BMU - Bar muscle up

MU - Muscle up (rings)

MASH - Massage, Active recovery, Stability hour (Active rest work)

CAL - Calorie

GHD - Glute hamstring developer

DB - Dumbell

TnG - Touch and go

session 1

Strength/skill:
front squats 4x4
back squats 4x4
WOD:
"angie"
100
pull-ups
push-ups
squats
sit-ups

session 2
Strength/skill:
EMOM: 6 min
power cleans x 3
3 burpees

WOD: part A
7 min AMRAP:
wallballs x8
kb swings x 10
o/h lunges x 12

 part B:
7 min AMRAP
HR push ups x10
 box jumps x8
 dips x6

session 3
Strength/skill:
pull ups 4 x 10
deadlifts 3x5

WOD
5 rounds for time:
thrusters x 10   40/30
200 meter sprint

session 4

strength/skill:
snatch prac
push press 5x3

WOD
AMRAP: 15 min
squat clean x 6 (60/40)
KTE x 8
slam ball x 10
pull ups x 12

session 5.

Strength/skill:
ring dips

EMOM: 6 min
pull ups x 5
burpees x 4

WOD:
21-15-9
KB snatches
box jumps
sit ups

session 6.

strength/skill
power clean 5x5

WOD:
front squats x 18
200 meter run
front squats x 12
400 meter run
front squats x 6
800 meter run
front squats x 4
broad jump 20 meters

session 7.

skill/strength:
split jerk prac
push jerk 4x4

WOD:
10-1
deadlift (1.5 bw)
burpee pull ups

sessions 8.

skill/strength:
muscle up prac
back squats 6x2 (@30x1 tempo)

WOD: 17 min AMRAP of

ground to overhead x1 (50/30)
sit ups x1
ground to overhead x2
sit ups x2
gound to over head x3
sit ups x3
etc…….

session 9

skill/strength:
max effort pull ups x3
kip practice

WOD: partner wod!
between the pair complete, one works one rests

200 squats
150 push ups

100 kb sumo high pulls (20/12)
50 burpees
50 wall balls

session 10

stregth/skill:
20 min to find 1RM power clean

EMOM: 10 min
KB clean and jerk x 4 Each arm
push ups x 10

WOD:
50-40-30-20-10
sit ups
double unders

session 11

EMOM: 5 min
front squat x 6 AHAP

WOD: chelsea!
EMOM 30 min
5 pull ups
10 push ups
15 squats

session 12

strength/skill:
strict press 3x5
push press 3x2

WOD:
10 burpees
100 m run
20 push ups
200 m run

40 push ups
300 m run
60 squats
400 m run
80 squats
500 m run
100 sit ups

session 13

strength/skill:
20 min to find 1RM deadlift

EMOM: 6 min
6 thrusters
2 burpees

WOD: TABATA
#1
sumo high pulls
push ups

1 min rest

#2
KB swings
T2B/kte

session 14
strength/skill:
back squat 3x5
push press 3x5

WOD: 5 rounds for time
power snatch x5
wall balls x10
o/h plate lunges x 15

session 15
stregth/ skill:

push press 3x5
muscle up practice

WOD: amrap 6 min

hang power snatch x 5 (40/25)
wallball x 10

session 16

strength/skill:
bar complex: x 5 rest 30 seconds after last movement
power clean/hang squat clean/push press x 2/back squat/ behind neck press.

WOD: 2 rounds
deadlift x 12   (120/70)
plate thrusters x 6   (20/10)
burpees x 12
box jumps x 18
burpees x 6
plate thrusters x 12
deadlifts x 6

session 17
strength/skill:
pistol squat practice
snatch balance

WOD
set clock for 15 min
run 800m
turkish get ups x5 each side
in remanding time: amrap of
12 pull ups
8 kb swings

session 18

strength/skill:

front squat 5 x 2 @ 20x1

EMOM 5 min
clean and press x 2 AHAP

WOD:
18-15-12-9-6
box jumps
sumo high pulls

session 19
strength/skill:
kb snatches from ground 3 x 3
deadlift 5 x 2

WOD:
100 squats
90 jumping lunges
80 push ups
70 kte
60 double unders
50 kb swings
40 pull ups
30 dips
20 burpees
10 muscle ups

session 20

strength/skill:
o/h squat 3x5

EMOM: 5 min
snatch x 1 AHAP

WOD: 21-15-9
push press (40/20)
KTE

session 21

strength/skill:
bent over rows 3 x 5

AMRAP 4 min
double unders

WOD:
200 m run
KB snatches x 21
sit ups x 15
HR push ups x 9
200 m run
sit up x 21
HR push ups x 15
KB snatches x 9
200 m run
HR push ups x 21
KB snatches x 15
sit ups x 9
100 m sprint

session 22

strength/skill:
ring pull ups with false grip, weighed if possible 4x5
rings dips weighted if possible 4x5

WOD:
AMRAP A: 7 min
burpee muscle ups x5
wall balls x 10

AMRAP B: 7 min
squat cleans x 6
hollow rocks x 12

session 23

strength/skill:
deadlifts 4x4
kb push press 4x4

EMOM 5 min
30 double unders
10 sit ups

WOD: 30-20-10
thrusters
box jumps

session 24
strength/skill:
front squats 5 5 4 2 1 1

EMOM: 6 min
7 pull ups
10 push ups

WOD: on the minute, add 3 reps to swings and 2 rep to sit ups till not reps not
completed in
minute.

kb swings x 3
sit ups x 2
kb swings x 6
sit ups x 4
kb swings x 9
sit ups x 6
kb swings x 12
sit ups x 8
kb swings x 15
sit ups x 10
kb swings x 18
sit ups x 12
kb swings x 21
sit ups x 14

session 25

strength/skill:
hand stand prac

EMOM: 8 min
EVEN : squat clean/hang power clean/ split jerk x 2
ODD : snatch grip high pulls x3

WOD: DIANE! 21-15-9
deadlifts (102/70)
handstand push ups

session 26
strength/skill:
muscle up prac
strict pull ups 3 x max effort

WOD:
squats x 100
push press x 10
squats x 80
push press x 8
squats x 60
push press x 6
squats x 40
push press x 4
squats x 20
push press x 2
squats x 10
push press x 1

session 27

strength/skill:
20 min to establish a 2RM back squat

EMOM: 5 min
clusters x 6
KTE x 6
WOD:
amrap for 12 min of

5 muscle ups/pull ups
10 push ups
15 wallballs

session 28

strength skill:
push press 5 x 2
behind neck press 3 x 3

WOD: amrap 10 min

power clean x 5
front squat x 10
push press x 15

session 29

strength skill:
OH squat 5x3
kipping/butterfly practice

WOD: 10-8-6-4-2
oh lunges 40/20
ring dips
double unders (100/80/60/40/20)

session 30

15 min to work on strength/skill weakness

death by burpee,

WOD: tabata
#1- power snatch
        sit ups

#2- kb swings
      plank

session 31
strength/skill:
front squat 3x6
strict press 3x6

WOD: AMRAP   15 min
complete as much as possible, add 5 reps to each movement per round
pull ups x 5
kb snatch x 5
push up x 5
pull ups x 10
kb snatch x 10
push up x10
pull ups x 15
kb snatch x 15
push ups x 15
etc……..

session 32

strength/skill:
clean and jerk 5x2

WOD:
3 rounds for time:
box jumps x 15

session 33

strength/skill:
max effort ring dips x3

WOD:
50 wallballs   (20/14)
5 muscle ups
40 KTE
4 muscle ups

30 thrusters (40/30)
3 muscle ups
20 burpees
2 muscle ups
10 HR push ups
1 muscle up

session 34

strength/skill:
back squat 4 x 10   @ 21X0

WOD: ROY
5 rounds for time:
deadlift x 15 (100/70)
box jumps x 20 (24/20)
pull ups x 25

session 35

strength/skill:
snatch balance 3x5

emom: 7 min
push ups x 15
sit ups x 10

WOD: 21/18/15
front rack lunges (50/30)
KB c+j each arm (16/12)

session 36

strength/skill:
pull ups (weighted/kipping/butterfly)

EMOM: 10
odd: squat clean x3 (60/40)

even: burpees x 10

WOD:
run 800 meters
kb sumo high pulls x 30
kb swings x 30
dips x 30
power cleans x 30 (30/20)
run 800 meters

session 37

strength/skill:
double unders 10 min

EMOM: 6min
split snatch x 2 AHAP

WOD: 3 x 3min AMRAP
#1
hollow rocks x 10
push ups x 10

rest 30 secs

#2
sit ups x 12
burpees x 7

rest 30 secs

#3
squats x 15
jumping lunges x 10

session 38
strength skill:
push press 3x3
push jerk 3x5

WOD: buy in: 20 burpees

amrap in 20 min

ground to overhead x 8 (50/35)
slam ball to shoulder x 16
pull ups x 24

Buy out: 20 burpees

session 39

strength/skill:
L- sit 3 x max effort hold

WOD:
3 rounds
Squats 75-50-25x
Pul-ups 50-35-20x
Ring dips 20-15-10x

session 40

strength/skill:
muscle up practice

emom: 6 min
squat snatch x 4
o/h squat x 4

WOD:
mary meets DT

AMRAP: 20 min

handstand push ups x5
pistol squats x 10 (alternating)

push ups x 15
deadlifts x12   (70/45)
hang power cleans x 9 (70/45)
push jerks x 6 (70/45)

session 41
strength/skill:
squat clean prac/ bar pull unders from toes
sumo high pulls 5 x 3

WOD:
double unders x 100
handstand push ups x 2
DU's x 80
HSPU x 4
DU's x 60
HSPU x 6
DU's x 40
HSPU x 8
DU's x 20
HSPU x 10

session 42

stregnth/skill:
front squats 4x3

EMOM: 5 min
behind the neck thrusters x 5
push ups x 10

WOD:
EMOM- 12 min
even: amrap of wall balls
odd: sit ups x 15

session: 43
strength/skill:
deadlift 5x5

WOD:

30 muscle ups for time
or 30 burpee pull ups

session 44

strength/skill:
power clean 3x3

EMOM: 6 min
double unders x 20
dips x 7

WOD: 2 x 4 min AMRAP
#1
O/H squat x 7
hollow rock x 10

1 min rest

#2
KB swings x 15
wall balls x 10

session 45

strength/skill:
back squat 6x2

WOD: partner chipper!
med ball sit ups x 60
burpees x 50 (1 for 1)
wall balls x 40 (1 throws 1 catch)
rusian twist x 30
toes to bar/KTE x 20 (1 for 1)
partner clap push ups x 10

session 46

strength/skill:

kipping/pull up prac

WOD:

5rft (25 min time cap)

squat cleans x 5   (60/40)
deadlift x 5 (120/80)
o/h plate lunges x 5 (20/10)

session 47

strength/skill:
20 min to establish 1rm snatch

Wod: EMOM 12 min
even: thrusters x 8
odd: amrap of jumping lunges

session 48

stregth/skill
strict press 3x5
push press 3x3

WOD: grace!
clean and jerk x 30 (60/40)

Session 50

Strength/ Skill:
Box Jump max Hight

WOD
5 rounds of:
15 wall balls

25 push ups
200 meter run

session 51

strength/skill:
back squats 4x4

EMOM: 6 min
clusters x 4
hollow rocks x 8

 WOD: amrap 8 min

KB snatch x 5 each arm (20/12)
hspu x 7
pull up x 9

session 52

strength/skill:
clean and jerk 5 x 3

WOD: 21-15-9
box jumps
shoulders to overhead

session 53

strength/skill:
front squat 3x6

 WOD:
 deadlift x 15 (100/70)
 cindy x 3

deadlift x 10
cindy x 2
deadlift x 5
cindy x 1

session 54

strength/skill:
thrusters 5x5

WOD:
wallballs x 100
pull ups x 50
sit ups x 100

session 55

strength/skill:
snatch touch and go 3x5

WOD: 15/12/9/6/3

front squat (60/40)
burpees

session 56

strength/skill:
pendlay rows 3x5

EMOM: 6 min
burpee pull ups x 6
toes to bar x 4

WOD:
4 rounds for time: 5 sit ups every 2 minutes

kb swings x 15
kb sumo high pulls x 15

kb snatch x 10 left arm
kb snatch x 10 right arm
kb thruster x 5 left
kb thruster x 5 right

session 57

strength/skill:
pull up prac, kip, butterfly

push ups on rings 3 x 12

WOD: AMRAP 5 min
ring dips x 20
in remainder timer
burpee broad jumps

1 min rest

AMRAP 5 min
pull ups x 20
in remainder time
walls balls

session 58

strength skill:
10 min to focus on a mobility weakness

WOD: filthy 50!

50 of each
box jumps
jumping pull ups
kb swings
walking lunges
KTE
push press (20/13)
back extensions
wall balls
burpees

double unders

session 59

strength/skill:
half hour to find deadlift 1rm

WOD: AMRAP 5min

hollow rocks x 12
double unders x 20

session 60

Strength/skill:
25 min to find push jerk 1 RM

WOD: with running clock complete-
in first 2 min AMRAP of KTE
then hold plank max effort.
score will be reps of KTE and seconds held in plank.

rest 1 min

WOD #2
same as above, replace KTE with sit ups

session 61

strength/skill:
30 min to find back squat 1rm

WOD: AMRAP 8min
push ups x12
sumo high pull x 8 (40/20)
bar facing burpees x 4

session 62

strength/skill:
turkish get ups 3 x 5 each arm
L-sit max effort hold x 3

WOD: 15/12//9/6/
power clean (60/40)
wall balls (20lbs/14lbs)

session 63

strength/skill:
20 meter farmers walk x 3

EMOM: 10 min
odd: hand release push ups x 10
even: no squat wall balls x 10

WOD: 5 RFT
kb racked walking lunges x20 meters.
pull ups x 20
ring dips x 20

session 64

strength/skill
OH squat   5-5-3-2-2

WOD: AMRAP 12 min
power snatch x 15 (30/20)
burpees x 7
T2B x 3

session 65

strength/skill:
muscle up 3x10

WOD The chief!

3 min AMRAP
power cleans x 3 (60/40)
push ups x 6
squats x 9
rest one minute

repeat for 5 cycles

session 66

strength/skill:
back squat
3 x 5 @ 80%-85% of 1RM

EMOM: 7 min
clusters x 3 (60/40)

WOD: 3RFT

plate thrusters x 18 (10/5)
hand stand push ups x 5

session 67

strength/skill:
strict press 4 x 3
push jerk 6 x 4 @ 60% 1RM

WOD:
goblet squats x 25
air squat hold 25 sec
goblet squat x 15
air squat hold 15 sec
goblet squat x 10
air squat hold 10 sec

goblet squat x 15
air squat hold 15 sec
goblet squat x 25
air squat hold 25 sec

session 68
strength/skill:
hand stand push ups 3 x max effort

EMOM: 6 min
clean + jerk (2+3) AHAP

WOD: 10 RFT
100m sprint
box jump x 5
rest 30 sec

session 69

strength/skill:
front squat 4x4 @ 85-90%
front squat 4 x 5 @ 60% 2-3-x-1

WOD: 4RFT
kb clean x 10 each arm
box jump x 15
kb swings x 25

session 70
strength/skill
weighted pull ups   4 x max effort
weighted dips   4 x max effort

WOD: 2RFT
deadlifts x 20 (60/40)
400 m
o/h squat x 20
T2B x20

push ups x 20
sumo high pull x 20 (60/40)

session 71
strength/skill
hang power clean 3 x 4

WOD: open work out 14.5 (25 min cap)
21/18/15/12/9/6/3

thrusters (40/30)
bar facing burpees

session 72

strength/skill:
snatch balance 5x3

WOD: buy in/out: 50 double unders or 200 single unders
o/h lunges x 20 (40/25)
strict pull ups x 25
box jumps x 30
strict pull ups x 25
o/h lunges x 20

session 73
strength/skill:
max effort push ups x 3

WOD: partner wod! AMRAP 20 min
25 MB sit-up/toss over 24″ box
20 Burpee / partner holds plank (no plank no rep)
15 Partner Squats (with a MB at your backs) MB falls out penalty 5 burpees
14/20#
10 Partner DL @65% of total body weight
* Your rep total is your score – total reps per round would be 50
* Partners may switch out burpees/plank hold as desired

session 74

strength/skill:
push press 5 x 5

WOD: half cindy
amrap 10 min
pull ups x 5
push ups x 10
squats x 15

session 75

strength skill:
hand stand push ups 3 x 10
T2B   3 x 10

WOD 1
AMRAP: 6 min
slam ball to shoulder x 7 (35/20)
slam ball on shoulder lunges 20 meters

WOD 2
AMRAP 6 min
wall balls x 10
man makers x 8

session 76

strength/skill:
deadlift 5 x 3 @ 90%

WOD: AMRAP 7min
push ups x 7
kb sumo high pulls x 9
KTE x 11

session 77

strength/skill:

rring rows 3x10

EMOM: 6 min
kb snatch x 5 EA
hollow rocks x 7

WOD: 5 rounds of
ME pull ups - 1 min
ME double unders - 1 min
ME toes to bar - 1 min
1 min rest

session 78

strength/skill:
push press 5 x 5

WOD: cindy
amrap 20 min
pull ups x 5
push ups x 10
squats x 15

session 79

strength/skill:
front squat 5 x 5

EMOM: 10 min
even-wall ball burpees x 8
odd- slam ball burpees x 6

WOD: 3RFT
thrusters x 8
sit ups x 16
kb swings x 24

session 80

strength/skill
bench press 5 x 5

WOD:
800 meter run
HR push ups x 20
400 meter run
ring dips x 20
200 meter run
burpees x 20
100 meter run

session 81

strength/skill:
emom- 10 min
even- power snatch-o/h squat x 2- hang squat snatch- o/h squat
odd-   snatch grip deadlift x 8,   3 burpees

snatch grip highpulls   4 x 4 AHAP

WOD: AMRAP 7 min
deadlift x 5 (100/60)
o/h plate lunges x 10 (20/10)
sit ups x 15

session 82

strength/skill:
20 min to find 3RM squat clean

WOD: barbara!
5 rft
20 pull ups
30 push ups
40 sit ups

50 squats
resting 3 min after each round

session 83

strength/skill:
back squat 5 x 5

back squat tempo 2-2-x-2 @ 70% of 1RM 5 x 3

WOD 21/15/9
kb swings
push press (40/30)

session 84

Strength/skill:
bench press 6 x 6

WOD AMRAP 12 min
power snatch x 6 (40/20)
burpee box jumps x 12
100 m run

session 85

strength/skill:
hang power snatch 5 x 4

EMOM- 5 min
squat x 15
push up x 10

WOD 10-1
burpee pull ups
wall balls

session 86
strength/skill:
pull ups (weighted/kipping/butterfly)

WOD - ANNIE
50-40-30-20-10
sit ups
double unders

session 87

strength/skill
front squat 4 x 6
strict press 4 x 6

WOD:
21/15/9
plate thrusters (20/10)
ring rows

session 88

strength/skill
pistol squats 3 x10 each leg

EMOM: 6min - 2 x power clean AHAP, push up x 10

WOD: AMRAP 12 min
muscle up x 5
sumo high pull x 7 (50/30)
KTE x 9
med ball clean x 11

session 89

strength/skill:
deadlift 5 x 5 @ 80-85%

WOD:
10-1 of dips with 20 meter broad jump between sets

session 90

strength/skill:
push press 3 x 5

EMOM 8 min- push jerk x 4

WOD: 2RFT
kb snatch left arm x 18 (20/12)
kb snatch right arm x 18
wall balls x 18
sit up x 18
double unders x 18 (50 singles)

session 91

strength/skill:
muscle up practice

WOD:
squat x 150
pull up x 30
squat x 100
pull up x 20
squat x 50
pull up x 10

session 92

strength/skill:
back squat 3x5

EMOM 6 min
clean and jerk x 3

WOD- AMRAP 12 min
slam ball x 6
ring push up x 12
push press x 6 (60/40)

session 93

strength/skill:
bench press 5x5 (heavier then last attempt)

WOD:
death by burpee
on the minute complete-
1 min- 1 burpee
2 min- 2 burpees
3 min - 3 burpees
complete until number of burpees in the minute is not achieved.

session 94

strength/skill:
pull ups max effort x 3 (rest as needed)

EMOM- 6 min
muscle snatch x 3

WOD- 3RFT
deadlift x 10 (120/70)
push up x 30
200 meter run

session 95

strength/skill:
O/H squat 5 x 5

WOD elizabeth!

21/15/9
clean (60/40)
ring dips

session 96

strength/skill:
hang power snatch 4-4-3-2-2-1-1

WOD 6 RFT
KTE x 6
wall ball x 6
sit up x 6

session 97
strength/skill:

Handstand Prac

WOD: 3 RFT
400 m run
kb swing x 30

session 98

strength/skill:
pendlay rows 4 x 6

med ball hip extension throws / plyometric throws (10 min)

WOD: AMRAP 7 min
power clean x 3 (60/40)
KTE x 3
power cleans x 5
KTE x 5
power cleans x 7
KTE x 7
etc.........

session 99

strength/skill:
tempo squats- 2-2-x-1 @50% 8x3 (30sec rest)

EMOM- 6 min
jump squats x 6 @ 30%

WOD:
pull up x 30
hollow rocks x 30
push up x 30
jumping lunges x 30
burpee x 30

session 100

strength/skill:
Split Jerk 6 x 2

WOD: 5RFT
wall balls x 20
broad jump 20 meters

session 101

strength/skill:
strict press 3 x 5
push jerk 3 x 3

3 x l-sit max effort

WOD: AMRAP 10 min
pull up x 1
push up x 1
pull up x 2
push up x 2
pull up x 3
push up x 3
etc......

session 102
strength/skill:
deadlift 75% x 2
then
60% 8x3 (90 sec rest)

WOD:
tabata - sit up
1 min rest
tabata - air squat
1 min rest
tabata - double unders

session 103

strength/skill:
kb snatch 5x3 AHAP

EMOM: 10 min
even - pistol squat x 10 alternating
odd -   double under x 20 (50 single)

WOD-   AMRAP - 7 min
power snatch x 5
pull up x 10

session 104

strength/skill:
o/h squat 3 x 5
front squat 3 x 5

WOD: EMOM 20 min
odd- clean and jerk (squat clean) x 2 AHAP
even- 30 sec max effort pull ups

session 105

strength/skill:

ring dips

WOD:
from 0-2 min
box jumps x 10
wall balls x 10

from 2-4 min
box jumps x 12
wall balls x 12

from 4-6 min
box jumps x 14
wall balls x 14

from 6-8 min
box jumps x 16
wall balls x 16
continue adding 2 reps per round until reps can't not be performed in allotted
time.

session 106

strength/skill:
pull up skill (kipping prac/butterfly)

WOD: 7 RFT

thrusters x 7   (40/30)
push ups x 7
kb c&j left arm x7 (20/12)
kb c&j right arm x 7
T2B x 7
sumo high pull x 7 (40/30)
deadlift x 7 (40/30)

session 107

strength/skill:
handstands

EMOM- 10 min
even - hang power clean x 3 AHAP
odd - plank 40 second

WOD AMRAP - 7 min

front squat x 5 (60/40)
kb swings x 15
double unders x 25 (60 singles)

session 108

strength/skill:
bench press 4x6

kb push press 3 x 4 each arm

WOD: AMRAP - 8 min
renegade rows x 10
slam ball burpees x 8

session 109

strength/skill:
back squat

WOD: 10 min AMRAP

burpees x 6
KTE x 8
air squat x 10

session 110

strength/skill:
deadlift x 2 @ 80%
then 8 x 3 @ 65% (90 secs rest)

WOD:
plate thruster tabata (20/10) (resting at bottom of squat)

rest 2 min
KTE tabata (hanging rest)
rest 1 min

3RFT
jumping lunge x 30
push up x 20

session 111

strength/skill:
snatch high pulls 5 x 3

hollow rocks 5 x 10

WOD: 4 x 3 min rounds

box over burpees x 15
kb swings x 20
max effort push ups in remainder time

rest 1 min

session 112

strength/skill:
strict press 3 x 5
push press 3 x 3

WOD:
6rft
clusters x 3 (60/40)
deadlifts x 4 (140/100)
burpees x 5

session 113

strength/skill:
20 min to find 1RM power clean

WOD: AMRAP 4 min

double unders x 20 (50 singles)
KB sumo high pull x 10 (20/12)

rest 1 min

AMRAP 4 min
push ups x 12
burpee pull ups x 6

session 114
strength/skill
front squat 8 x 3 @ 85-90%

WOD: 3 RFT
box overs with med ball x 20 (20/14)
wall balls x 10
sit ups with med ball x 5

session 115
strength/skill:
ring rows 4 x 10
ring push ups 4 x10

WOD: AMRAP 15 min

200 m run
sit ups x 10
box dips x 15
walking lunge x 20

session 116

strength/skill:
snatch 5 x 3 @ 80-85%

WOD: 4RFT

squat clean x 6 (50/35)
thrusters x 8
bar facing burpees x 6

session 117
strength/skill:
bench press
20 min to find 1RM

WOD: 10 - 1
slam ball to shoulder
front rack lunges (50/35)

session 118
strength/skill:
muscle up 3 x 5 (or band assisted)

WOD: Fran!
21/15/9
thrusters (43/30)
pull ups

session 119
strength/skill:
pendlay rows 5 x 5

WOD: for time
buy in/out: 50 double unders/120 singles
150 squats
100 push ups
50 sit ups
 3 burpees @ every 2 minute mark

session 120

strength/skill:
deadlift 85% x 2
then 70% 6x3 (90 secs rest)

WOD: AMRAP 8 min
hspu x 6
c & J x 8 (50/35)
hollow rocks x 10

session 121

strength/skill:
strict pull ups 3 x 5-10 @ 31x2

rope ascends

WOD: tabata
plate snatches

rest 1 min

AMRAP 9 min
buy in- 70 double unders (150 singles)
3 wall balls
3 KTE
6 wall balls
6 KTE
9 wall balls
9 KTE
etc…..

session 122

strength/skill:
hang squat clean 5 x 3

EMOM 10 min
even- front squat x 2, push press, split jerk
odd- strict knees to elbows x 7

WOD AMRAP- 7 min
push ups x 2
kbshp x 2
push ups x 4
kbshp x 4
push ups x 6
kbshp x 6
etc….

session 123

strength/skill:
back squat- 60% x 3, 70% x 3, 80% x max, 70% x 4, 60% x 4

WOD: quad tabata
double unders
power snatch
box jumps
sit ups

session 124

strength/skill:
rope ascends

EMOM 8 min
even- hollow rocks x 12
odd- pistol squats x 5 each legs

WOD:
kb snatch r/a x 9
kb snatch l/a x 9
pull ups x 21
kb snatch r/a x 15
kb snatch l/a x 15
pull ups x 15
kb snatch r/a x 21
kb snatch l/a x 21
pull ups x 9

session 125
strenghth/skill:
ring dips 3 x max effort
hanging L-sit max effort x 3

WOD:
buy in- power clean x 12 (70/40)
3 Rounds
burpees x 12
hspu x 12
buy out- wall ball x 12

session 126

strength/skill:
deadlift 90% x 2
then
75% 5 x 3 reps (90 sec rest)

WOD: AMRAP 7 min
renegade rows x 8
broad jump x 20 m
ring rows x 8
broad jump x 20 m

session 127

strength/skill:
strict press 3 x 5
push press 3 x 3
push jerk 3 x 1

WOD:
18/15/12
plate thrusters (20/10)
200 m run

session 128

strength/skill
bench press 4 x 6reps @85%

WOD: clock set for 10 min
2 rounds of
double unders x 50 (150 singles)
wallballs x 15
sit ups x 15
in remainder time AMRAP
burpee pull ups

session 129

strength/skill:
power clean 5 x 3 @ 80-85%

WOD: 3 x 3min rounds
box jumps x 20
squat jump x 8 (30/20)
remainder time AMRAP of box dips

Session 130

strength/skill:
10 min on mobility weakness
10 min kipping/butterfly/bar muscle up prac

WOD:
hollow rocks x 80
push ups x 70
squats x 60
kb snatches x 50 (25 each arm) (20/12)
sit ups x 40
deadlift x 30 (50/30)
squat clean x 20
power clean x 10

session 131

strength/skill:
front squat 6 x 2 @ 90-95%

WOD: 18/15/12/9
shoulder to overhead (40/30)
KTE

session 132

strength/skill:
farmers walk 3 x 20m AHAP

EMOM- 8 min

power snatch x 2 AHAP
med ball clean x 8

WOD
AMRAP- 3 min
kb cleans x 6 E/A
hollow rocks x 8

rest 1 min

AMRAP- 2 min
kb snatches x 6 E/A
jumping lunges x 10

rest 1 min

AMRAP 1 min
burpees

session 133

strength/skill:
handstand

EMOM- 8 min
odd- dips x 7, deficit push ups x 5
even- wallballs x 15

WOD- AMRAP 10 min

wall walks x 3
pull ups x 5
double unders x 20 (60 singles)

session 134

strength/skill:
push press 5 x 3 @ 80-85%

WOD- open work out 12.4
complete as many reps/rounds as possible in 12 min of-

150 wall balls
90 double unders
30 muscle ups

session 135

strength/skill:

accumulate 3 min of l-sit hold from bar

EMOM- 6 min
power snatch x 2, o/h squat x 2

WOD- 3 RFT
med ball clean x 30
burpees x 20
KTE x10

session 136

strength/skill:
deadlift 90% x 2
then 75% 5 x 3 reps (90 secs rest)

WOD- AMRAP 7 min
deficit push ups x 10 (6"/3")
strict pull ups x 5
kb swings x 10 (20/12)

session 137

strength/skill:
bench press- 5 x 5 @ 85%

2 RFT (3 burpees at every 2min mark)
plate snatch x 40 (20/10)
hollow rock x 30
plate thruster x 20
sit up x 10

session 138

strength/skill:
pause front squat 8 x 3 reps @60%
first set 3 sec pause, second set - 4 sec, third set - 5 sec....etc

WOD- AMRAP 10 min
thrusters x 9 (50/35)
double unders x 18 (60 singles)
bar over burpees x 9

session 139

strength/skill:
dips 3 x 10 (weighted if possible)
pull ups 3 x10 (weighted if possible)

WOD: 10 x 1 min rounds

deadlift x 3 (1.5 bw)
50m sprint
burpees in remainder
rest 2 min

session 140

strength/skill:
hang snatch 7 x 2

WOD- AMRAP 7 min

kb push press x 5 each arm (20/12)
kb lunge x 10 (alternating)
kb swing x 15

session 141

strength/skill:
deadlift 3 x 3 @ 80% then

3 x 3 @65% (90 sec rest)

WOD- 10-8-6-4-2
thrusters (50/35)
burpee pull ups

session 142
strength/skill:
o/h squat 6 x 4

EMOM 7 min
ring push ups x 10
hollow rocks x 8

WOD 7 min AMRAP
wall ball x 10
kb swing x 10 (20/16)
box jumps x 10

session 143
strength/skill:
muscle up

WOD: 12 min running clock
clean and jerk x 20 (30/20)
pull ups x 20
clean and jerk x 15 (40/30)
pull ups x 15
clean and jerk x 10 (50/35)
pull ups x 10
remainder time amrap of clean and jerk (60/40)

session 144

strength/skill
pendlay rows 5 x 5

WOD:12 min running clock
squat clean x 1 (60/40)
sit up x 1
jumping lunges x 10

squat clean x 2
sit up x 2
jumping lunges x 20

squat clean x 3
sit up x 3
jumping lunges x 30
etc…….

session   145

strength/skill:
back squat 7 x 2 @ 95%

WOD: 15/12/9/6/3
handstand push ups
sumo high pull (50/35)

session 146

strength/skill:
pull ups

EMOM- 8 min
20 meter pinch grip plate walk (20/10)
8 burpees

WOD- AMRAP 10 min

box overs x 8
ring dips x 10
rope climb x 1

session 146

strength/skill:

bar complex- (power clean/press x2/cluster) x 5 AHAP rest as needed

WOD:
21/15/9
deadlift (100/70)
kb snatch (20/12)

1 min rest

1 min amrap of hollow rocks

session 147

strength/skill:
bench press 5 x 3

WOD-
Tabata each with 30 sec rest between each tabata

wall ball
box jump
hollow rock
burpee

session 148

strength/skill:
L-sit accumulate 3 min

ring dips 3 x 8

WOD 12 min ascending ladder amrap

3 front squats
3 jumping pull ups

6 front squats
6 jumping pull ups

9 front squats
9 jumping pull ups

etc....

session   149

strength/skill:
strict press 4 x 8

WOD: for time   (buy in/out 30 sit ups)
100 m run
kb swing x 10 (20/16)
200 m run
KB walking lunge x 20
200 m run
kb swing x 10
100 m run

session 150

strength/skill:
snatch- 20 min to find 1RM

WOD:
toes to bar x 40
o/h squat x 15 (40/30)
T2B x 30
o/h squat x 12
T2B x 20
o/h squat x 10

session 151

strength/skill:
pistol squats 3 x 10 each leg

EMOM: 8 min
odd- power clean x 2 @ 90%
even- hollow rocks x 15

WOD: amrap 4 min
wall balls x 7
kb swings x 7
push ups x 7

rest 1 min

amrap 3 min
kbshp x 8
pull up x 4
burpee x 2

session 152

strength/skill:
deadlift 85% x 2
75% 3 x 3

WOD AMRAP 7 min

20m ball throw (35/20)
20m walking lunge (ball on shoulder)

session 153

strength/skill:
split jerk- 5 x 1

WOD: 4 RFT
double unders x 30
sit ups x 20
thrusters x 10 (50/35)

session 154

strength/skill:
power clean- 20 min to find a heavy double

emom- 5 min- fr lunges x 6 each leg (40/30)

WOD: AMRAP 10 min

burpee muscle up x 3
front squats x 5 (60/40)
hspu x 7

session 155

strength/skill:
ring push ups 3 x 10 (deficit if possible)
ring rows 3 x 15

WOD- AMRAP 12 min
slam ball burpees x 10 (35/20)
goblet squat x 15 (20/12)
wall ball x 20
run 200m

session 156

strength/skill:
back squat 6 x 3 @ 85-90%
front squat- 5 x 3 - 23x1 @ 50% (30 sec rest)

WOD- AMRAP 6 min
ground to overhead x 5 (50/35)
bar over burpee x 20

session 157

strength/skill:
muscle up

WOD: pyramid wod!
3/6/9/12/15/12/9/6/3

KB swings (20/12)
ring dips
hollow rocks

(200 meter run before the 12 rep rounds)

session 158

strength/skill:
L-sit accumulate 3 min

WOD: 8 x 2 min round
pull up x 5
push up x 10
squat x 15
pull up x 5
push up x 10
squat x 15

sit ups in remainder time
1 min rest

session 159

strength/skill:
deadlift x 2 @ 90%
3 x 3 @ 75% (90 sec rest)

WOD: 3 rounds for time

shoulder to overhead x 12 (40/30)
rope climb x 3

session 160
strength/skill:
toes to bar 3 x 8-10

WOD-
5 rounds for time
pull up x 20
push up x 20
squat x 20
sit up x 20
deadlift x 20 (40/30)

session   161

strength/skill:
bench press- 5 x 5

WOD: 6 x 2min rounds
ring rows x 8
hollow rocks x 10
jumping lunge x 12 (6 each leg)
max effort wall balls in remainder time

session 162

strength/skill: 25 min to find heaviest complex of:

power clean/hang power clean/ high hang power clean/ jerk

WOD: AMRAP 8 min
box jumps x 12
power snatch x 6 (40/30)
burpee x 3

session 163

strength/skil:
front squat- 6 x 3

WOD- AMRAP 5 min
double under x 20
plate thruster x 10 (20/10)

1 min rest

AMRAP- 5 min
KTE x 7
push up x 14

session 164
strength/skill:
mobility work

WOD: helen
3 rounds for time
400 m run
21 kb swings
12 pull ups

session 165

strength/skill:
strict press 3 x 5
push press 3 x 3

WOD: 10 min running clock
2 min amrap of each
cluster (60/40)
wallball (20/14)
double unders
muscle ups
burpee broad jumps

session 166
stregth/skill:
deadlift 95% x 2
            70 % 3 x 3 (90 sec rest)

WOD: 4 rounds
toes through rings x 7
kb snatch x 16 (8 each arm)
100 m run

session 167

strength/skill:
kb push press 5 x 3

WOD: for time

burpee x 10
400 m run

ring push up x 20
200 m run
ring row x 20
200 m run
push up x 20
200 m run
pull up x 20
400 m run
burpee x 10

session 168

strength/skill:
back squat 6 x 4 @ 85-90%

EMOM 6 min
jumping squats x 5 @ 30%

WOD- 30/20/10
kb clean + press (15/10/5 each arm 20/12)
pull up

session 169

strength/skill:
snatch balance 5 x 3

WOD: AMRAP 20 min
clean and press x 2 (70/45)
deadlift x 4
bar facing burpee x 6
toes to bar x 8
box jump x 10
push up x 12

session 170

strength/skill:
strict pull ups 4 x 7 (weighted if >7 is achievable)

WOD: complete until failure

0-2 min: rope ascend x 2
          front squat x 2 (50/35)

2-4 min: rope ascend x 2
          front squat x 4

4-6 min: rope ascend x 2
          front squat x 6
etc……

session 171

strength/skill:
bench press 6 x 2

WOD: for time
100 burpees
(perform 2 hang power clean @ 70/40 emom)
12 min cap

session 172

strength/skill:
overhead squats 3 x 5

EMOM-7 min:
KB snatch from ground x 3 EA

WOD: 7 min ascending ladder
1 of each, 2 of each, 3 of each etc…
wall balls
sit ups

session 173

strength/skill:
thrusters- find 3RM

WOD: AMRAP 15 min
deadlift x 1 (120/80)
squat x 30

box jump x 20
dips x 10
200 m run

session 174

strength/skill:
handstand prac

WOD: 10-1
toes to bar
push ups

2 min rest

10-1
pull ups
squats

session 175
strength/skill:
find 1RM back squat

WOD: amrap 6 min

hang power snatch x 5 (40/25)
wallball x 10

session 176

strength/skill:
clean 5 x 2

WOD: tabata
#1- sumo high pulls (40/30)
        push ups

#2- hollow rocks
        bar over burpees

session 177

strength/skill:
muscle up prac

WOD:
buy in: 50 squats

3 rounds
box over with ball on shoulder x 8 (35/20)
cluster x 10 (40/30)

buy out: 100 double under

session 178

strength/skill: bear complex
power clean/front squat/push press/ back squat/ push press.
perform 7 times without putting bar down. Find heaviest complex in 5 rounds

WOD: AMRAP 7 min
burpee pull up

session 179

strength/skill:
L-sit 3 x max effort hold

WOD: Deck of cards team wod!
25 min cap
red # card = pull ups
black # card = thrusters (40/30)
face cards j,q,k = 10 bar over burpees
joker = 5 deadfall cleans (35/20)

team with most cards at end of 25min wins!

session 180

strength/skill:
skin the cat

EMOM: 6 min
dead ball clean x 5
dead ball squat x 5

WOD: fran
21/15/9
thrusters
pull ups

session 181

strength/skill:
pendlay rows 5 x 5

toes to bar/ KTE 5 x 10

WOD: 7 rounds
two arm swing x 1 (20/12)
one arm swing x 1 left
one arm swing x 1 right
kb c+j left x 1
kb c+j right x1
kb snatch x 1 left
kb snatch x 1 right
burpee x 1

add one rep to each movement each round

session   182

strength/skill:
deadlift 5 x 3

WOD: AMRAP 15 min

ground to over head x 2 (40/30)
100 m run
G2O x 4
200 m run

G2O x 6
300 m run
G2O x 8
400 m run
G2O x 10
500 m run
etc.......

session   183

strength/skill:
bench press 5 x 5

WOD: for time

box jump x 40
hollow rock x 30
pull up x 20
hand stand push up x 10
muscle up x 10
pull up x 20
hollow rock x 30
box jump x 40

session 184

strength/skill:
front squat 5 x 5
paused front squat 3 x 3 (3 sec pause)

WOD: AMRAP- 7 min
sumo high pull x 7 (50/35)
hspu x 9

session   185

strength/skill:
handstand prac

WOD: AMRAP 7 min
wall ball x 12

kb swing x 12
50 m sprint

1 min rest

AMRAP 7 min
kb sumo high pull x 10
HR push up x 8
jumping lunge x 10

TABATA
hollow rock

session 186

strength/skill:
power snatch 5 x 3

WOD: 4 Rounds for time
ring dips x 15
sit up x 20
double under x 25

session 187

strength/skill:
push ups - 1 min max effort

WOD: 8 x 1 min round
squat clean x 2 (80/50)
bar over burpee in remainder of minute

90 sec rest

session 188

strength/skill:
pull ups 4 x max effort (Strict)
ring rows 4 x 10

WOD: nancy
5 rounds for time

400 m run
15 x o/h squat (40/30)

session 189

strength/skill:
deadlift find 1 RM

WOD: 18 min running clock
run 1.6km
remaining time complete amrap of cindy (5 pull ups, 10 push ups, 15 squats)

session 190

strength/skill:
strict press 5 x 3

EMOM: 6 min
hang squat clean x 2 AHAP

WOD: AMRAP 10 min
burpee box jump x 8
power clean x 4 (60/40)
plyo push ups x 10 (6"/3" jump)

session   191

strength/skill:
back squat 5 x 5

WOD: AMRAP 10 min

pull up x 7
med ball clean x 9
sit up x 11

session 192

strength/skill:
o/h squat- 5 x 3

EMOM - 7 min
o/h lunge x 8 (AHAP)

WOD- 3 rounds for time

hang power clean x 6 (60/40)
wall ball x 12
push up x 18

session 193

strength/skill:
muscle up

WOD: 3 rounds for time

deadlift x 4 (140/90)
kb push press x 5 each arm (24/16)
dead ball clean x 6 (35/20)
muscle up x 7
hspu x 8
kb lunge x 9 Each leg
box jump x 10
double under x 75

session 194

strength/skill:
split jerk 5 x 1

WOD:
AMRAP - 5 min
kb clean x 6 each arm (20/16)
pull up x 6

1 min rest

AMRAP - 5 min

double under x 30
sit up x 10

session 195

strength/skill:
front squat 5 x 3
paused front squats 5 x 1 AHAP (3 sec pause)

WOD:18/12/6/12/18
kb thruster (20/12)
dips

session 196

strength/skill:
handstand (headstand hold, wall walk, freestanding)

turkish get up 3 x each side

WOD: AMRAP 10 min
buy in: 20 hollow rocks

knees to elbow x 2
wall ball x 2
sumo high pull x 3 (50/35)

kte x 4
wall ball x 4
sumo high pull x 3

kte x 6
wall ball x 6
sumo high pull x 3

etc….

session 197

strength/skill:
bench press 6 x 2

WOD: AMRAP 12 min
100 m run
squats x 10
burpees x 10

200 m run
squats x 20
burpees x 10

300m run
squats x 30
burpees x 10

400 m run
squats x 40
burpees x 10

session 198

strength/skill: find heaviest complex of-
power clean/ squat clean/ hang squat clean

EMOM 5 min
snatch grip sumo high pull AHAP

WOD: Karen
150 wall balls for time

session 199

strength/skill:
pull up

WOD: AMRAP 15 min
hspu x 5
T2B x 10
med ball clean x 15

session   200

strength/skill:
L-sit 3 x max effort

WOD: partner 200!

in pairs complete AMRAP in 30 min

200 push ups
200 pull ups
200 squats
200 burpees
break up as needed
(200m run at every 5 min mark)

session 201

strength/skill:
push jerk TnG 5 x 3

EMOM- 7 min
power snatch x 2
o/h squat x1

3 RFT
thruster x 7 (50/35)
dips x 10
rope ascend

session 202

strength/skill:
pendlay rows 5 x 5

WOD: for time
double unders x 50
front squats x 21   (50/35)
plyo push ups x 9 (6"/3")

double unders x 50
front squats x 15
plyo push ups x 15

double unders x 50
front squats x 9
plyo push ups x 21

session 203

strength/skill:
find heaviest complex of- push press to split jerk

WOD: 6 RFT
100 m walk with plate over head (20/10)
double under x 75

session 204

strength/skill:
back squat 7 x 3

WOD: AMRAP - 7 min
cluster x 6 (60/40)
box jump x 8 (30/24)

session 203

strength/skill:
hang power clean 5 x 4

WOD: for time
1 mile run
pull ups x 30
200m run
pull ups x 30
1 mile run

session 204

strength/skill:
strict toes to bar/KTE 4 x 10

WOD: "air force"

thrusters x 20 (40/30)
sumo high pulls x 20
push jerks x 20
o/h squat x 20
front squat x 20

4 burpees emom

session 205

strength/skill:
bench press 6 x 3

WOD: AMRAP 7 min
hollow rock x 10
burpee pull up x 7

session 206

strength/skill:
deadlift 5 x 3

WOD: AMRAP 8 min
thrusters (20/15)
5 burpees emom

session 207

strength/skill:
muscle up

WOD: 21/15/9
wall balls
push up
toes to bar/ KTE

rest 5 min

Tabata
alternate hollow rock / plank

session   208

strength/skill:
overhead squat 5 x 5

WOD: for time
box jump x 50
push up x 50
double under x 50
jumping lunge x 50
shoulder to overhead x 50 (30/20)

session 209
strength/skill:
emom 12 min
odd- 5 x power snatch
even-   max effort pull up in 30 sec

WOD: 3 RFT
400 m run
kb snatch x 7 each arm (20/12)
rope ascend x 1

session 210

strength/skill:
strict press 4 x 6

EMOM 8 mn
push jerk x 2 AHAP

WOD: AMRAP 5 min
deadlift x 1 (150/100)
broad jump x 20 meters

rest 2 min

AMRAP 5 min
squat clean x 1 (90/50)
push up x 30

session 211

strength/skill:
emom 12 min
odd- 5 x power snatch
even-   max effort pull up in 30 sec

WOD: 3 RFT
400 m run
kb snatch x 7 each arm (20/12)
rope ascend x 1

session 212

strength/skill:
overhead squat 5 x 5

WOD: for time
box jump x 50
push up x 50
double under x 50
jumping lunge x 50
shoulder to overhead x 50 (30/20)

session 213

strength/skill:
paused front squat 5 x 4

WOD: 10 min fran ladder

10 min amrap of:
 pull up x 2
thruster x 2   (40/30)

pull up x 4
thruster x 4

pull up x 6
thruster x 6

etc……

session 214

strength/skill:
find clean and jerk 1rm

WOD: AMRAP 7 min

kb swing x 15
hollow rock x 10
burpee x 5

session 215

remembrance day hero wod

HAMMER
 5 rounds
power clean x 5 (60/40)
front squat x 10
push jerk x 5
pull up x 20

rest 90 sec

session 216

strength/skill:
bench press
20-10-8-5-5-5-10

WOD: 5 rounds for time

100 m sprint
pull up x 10
100 m sprint
burpee x 10

30 sec rest

session 217

strength/skill:
deadlift 6 x 2

WOD: 3 rft

wall ball x 21
handstand push up x 15
sumo high pull x 9 (50/35)

session 218

strength/skill:
ring dips 5 x 5-10 (if more then 10 is achievable add weight)

WOD: 5 rft

double under x 50
air squat x 25
squat snatch x 5 (40/30)

session 219

strength/skill:
back squat 3 x 3
front 3 x 3

WOD: AMRAP 15 min

in pairs
partner 1 holds deadlift (100/70)
partner 2 performs 15 burpees. (burpees only count wilst bar is being held)
swap

partner 1 holds kb in goblet squat position
partner 2 performs 20 jumping lunges (lunges only count if goblet squat is

below parallel)
swap

partner 1 holds plate over head (20/10)
partner 2 performs 20 pushups. (push ups only count if plate is overhead)
swap

session 220

strength/skill:
snatch 5 x 2

WOD: AMRAP 10 min
bear complex x 3 (50/35)
100 m run
kb snatch x 3 each arm (20/12)
200 m run

session 221

strength/skill:
L- sit hold 3 x max effort
muscle up prac

WOD:
buy in/out: 30 wall balls
3 rounds
burpee box jump x 10
squat clean x 8 (60/40)

session   222

strength/skill:
back squat- 20/10/8/5/5/5

WOD: AMRAP 4 min
hollow rock x 10
double under x 25

rest 1 min

AMRAP 4 min
push up x 15
100 m run

session 223

strength/skill
pull up 4 sets (5-10 rep range, add weight if possible)
dips 4 x 5-10

WOD: 10 rounds for time

muscle up x 3
plate snatch x 6 (20/10)

session 224

strength/skill:
strict press 3 x 5
push press/push jerk 3 x 3 + 1

WOD: 3 rounds for time
toes to bar x 30
thrusters x 15 (40/30)

session 225

strength/skill:
EMOM - 12 min
even- deadlift x heavy 4
       push up x 10
odd- 30 sec max effort jumping lunge

WOD: 12 x 90 sec rounds

50m sprint
5 burpees
max effort wall balls
rest 45 seconds

session   226

strength/skill:
front rack lunges 4 x 12m walk

WOD: AMRAP - 12 min
hang power clean x 6 (60/40)
pull up x 12
squat x 18

session 226

strength/skill:
bench press find 2RM

WOD- 27/21/18/15
T2B
KB swings (20/16)
EMOM 4 burpees

session 227

strength/skill:
thruster 5 x 3

WOD:
amrap- 10 min

o/h squat x 8 (40/30)
double under x 25

session 228

strength/skill:
handstand

WOD: elizebeth
21/15/9
clean (60/40)
ring dips

rest 2 min

800m run

session 229

strength/skill:
back squat 5 x 5
jump squat @ 40% of above (6 reps emom - 6 min)

WOD
3 rounds for time
400m run
clean n jerk x 20 (40/30)

session 230
strength/skill:
turkish get up 3 x 3 each arm

WOD: partner wod

20 min running clock

partner 1 runs 200m with med ball
partner 2 performs amrap of thrusters (30/20)
swap

partner 1 skips 150 skips
partner 2 performs amrap of slam ball over shoulder (35/20)
swap

partner 1 runs 200m with med ball
partner 2 performs amrap of pullups/ring rows

swap

partner 1 skips 150 skips
partner 2 performs amrap of wall balls
swap

go back to start

session 231

strength/skill:
deadlift 6 x 3 @ 85-90%

WOD: 7 round for time
pull up x 7
push up x 7
squat x 7
jumping lunge x 7

session 232

strength/skill:
30 min running clock

0-10 min: clean and jerk every 30 secs @ 55%
10-20 min: c+j every 30 sec @ 70%
21-25 min: c+j x 2 @ 80 %
26-30 min: c+j x 1 @ 85@

WOD: for time
burpees x 50

session 233

strength/skill:
O/H squats 5 x 3 (2-3-x-0 tempo)

WOD:
o/h squat x 30 (30/20)
handstand push up x 20
o/h squat x 20
hspu x 15

o/h squat x 10
hspu x 10

session 234

strength/skill:
4 attempts at complex- KTE/T2B/pull up/ C2B
and/or pull up - 4 x max effort strict

WOD AMRAP - 10 min
box jump x 20 (24/20)
double under x 75 (200 singles)

rest 2 min

tabata- hollow rock

session 235

strength/skill:
bench press 5 x 5

WOD: AMRAP - 15 min
ascending ladder
turkish get up x 1 Each arm (16/10)
squat clean x 1 (70/50)

turkish get up x 2 Each arm
squat clean x 2

increase 1 rep each set till 12 min expires

session 236

strength/skill:
handstand hold 4 x 30 secs
strict toes to bar/knees to elbow/knee tuck 3 x 10

WOD: buy in: 100 double unders (200 singles)

4 rounds
push up x 15
deadlift x 10 (80/50)
pate snatch x 5 (20/15)

buy out: 30 hollow rocks

session 237
strength/skill: emom- 10 min
full clean/hang clean/power clean

WOD:
21/15/9/6/3

shoulder to overhead (50/35)
pull up

session 238
strength/skill:
find front squat 1rm

WOD:
AMRAP- 12 min

rope climb x 2
push up x 20
400 m run

session 239

strength/skill:
muscle up

WOD: 2 rounds for time

deadlift x 24 (110/70)
box jump x 24
wall ball x 24
bar over burpees x 24
wall ball x 24

box jump x 24
power clean x 24 (50/35)

session 240

strength/skill:
ring row 4 x 10-15
ring push up 4 x 10-15

WOD: 5 rounds for time

o/h lunges x 12 (40/30)
hspu x 8

session 241
strength/skill:
back squat 7 x 2

WOD:
22/16/10
hang snatch (40/30)
wall ball

session 242

strength/skill:
bench press- 3 x 20

WOD: death by front squat @ 60% BW
              death by sumo high pull @ 50% BW
              death by burpee

session 243

strength/skill:
pull up 5 x 5 (weighted if possible)
dips 5 x 5 (weighted if possible)

WOD: AMRAP 10 min
TTB x 12

100 meter med ball carry (20/14)
hollow rock x 12

session 244

strength/skill:

shoulder to overhead - find 1 rm
then 3 x 8 @65-70% of above (90 sec rest)

WOD: for time

complex squat clean/thruster x 10 (40/30) (must squat out of clean THEN re-squat for the thruster)
800m run
same complex as above x 10

session 245

strength/skill:
hang snatch - 3 x 4
snatch grip deadlift 3 x 4

WOD: 15-5
KB swing (24/16)
push up

session 246
last WOD for the year!

12 days of xmas!
complete 1, then 2,1,   then 3,2,1, then 4,3,2,1 until you complete all 12

1- squat clean (50/35)
2- hspu
3- front squat
4- sumo high pull

5- C2B pull ups
6- box jumps
7- burpees
8- push ups
9- wall balls
10- kb swings (20/12)
11- deadlifts
12- thrusters

OR

1- cluster
2 - front squat
3 - hang power clean
4 - push jerk
5 - deadlift
6 - bar over burpee
7 - push ups
8 - wallballs
9 - sit ups
10 - TTb
11 - thrusters
12 - front rack lunges

session 247

strength/skill:
back squat 4 x 10

WOD: 3 rft

wallball x 20
burpee x 15
lunge x 10 (each leg)

session 248

strength/skill:
strict press 4 x 10

WOD: AMRAP 10 min
push up x 10
pull up x 9

hollow rock x 8
kte x 7

session 249

strength/skill:
power clean 5 x 3

WOD: 21/15/9
squat clean (50/35)
box jump

session 250

strength/skill:
deadlift 4 x 8

WOD: for time

run 400m
push press x 21 (50/35)
plate snatch x 10 (20/15)

run 200m
push press x 15
plate snatch x 10

run 100m
push press x 9
plate snatch x 10

session 251

strength/skill:
EMOM- 21 min
1- o/h lunge x 7 (each leg) 20/10 plate
2- burpee x 12
3- C+J x 3 (70/45)

WOD: for time
thrusters x 25 (40/30)
sit up x 40

thrusters x 25

session 252

strength/skill:
double unders 10 min

WOD: 3 x 3min AMRAP
#1
hollow rocks x 10
push ups x 10

rest 30 secs

#2
sit ups x 12
burpees x 7

rest 30 secs

#3
squats x 15
jumping lunges x 10

session 253   12/1/15

strength skill:
push press 3x3
push jerk 3x5

WOD: buy in: 20 burpees

20 min amrap

ground to overhead x 8 (50/35)
slam ball to shoulder x 16
ring dips x 24

session 254

stregnth/skill:
Deadlift: find 1rm

EMOM: 5 min
behind the neck thrusters x 5
push ups x 10

WOD: 15 min amrap
pull ups x 10
burpees x10
kte x 10

session 255

Strength/ Skill:
Box Jump max Hight -15 min

WOD: 5 RFT
15 wall balls
50 d/u or 100 singles
200 meter run

session 256

strength/skill:
Bench press: 3x10

WOD: The chief!

3 min AMRAP
power cleans x 3 (60/40)
push ups x 6
squats x 9
rest one minute

repeat for 5 cycles

session 257
strength/skill
weighted pull ups   4 x max effort
weighted dips   4 x max effort

WOD: 2RFT
deadlifts x 20 (50/35)
400 m run
o/h squat x 20 (50/35)
T2B x20
push ups x 20
sumo high pull x 20 (50/35)

session 258

strength/skill:
front squat 5 x 5

WOD:
3 rounds for total reps of:
1 min push ups
1 min kb swings
1 min air squats
1 min hollow rocks
1 min hang power clean (50/35)
 1 min rest

session 259

strength/skill:
overhead squat 5 x 3

WOD: filthy 50

50 of each
box jump (24/20)
jumping pull ups
kettlebell swings (16/12)
walking lunge
KTE
push press (20/13)
wallball
burpee
double under

session 260

strength/skill:

EMOM: 7 min
power clean/ 2 x front squat

EMOM: 7 min
hang squat clean/ front squat

EMOM: 7 min
full clean

rest 2 min between each emom.

WOD: 10 min ascending ladder
burpee pull up
thruster

session   261

strength/skill:
split jerk 6 x 1

WOD: 3 rft
21 x kb swing (20/16)
15 x sit ups
9 x double unders

rest 1 min (clock still running)

6 rounds
deadlift x 10 (50/35)
push up x 10

session 262

strength/skill:
L- sit hang 3 x max effort

WOD: fran
21/15/9
thrusters (42.5/30)

pull ups

rest 3 min

tabata hollow rock
rest 1 min
tabata thruster (20/13)

session 263

strength/skill:
muscle up prac

WOD: 12 min running clock

power snatch x 35 (30/20)
burpee x 35
KTE x 35
max effort wall ball

session 264

strength/skill:
deadlift 5x5

WOD: 5 RFT
box jump x 9
kb sumo high pull x 12 (20/16)
400 m run

session 265

Aus day hero WOD!

BLAKE: 4 rounds for time

100 ft overhead walking lunge (20/13)
30 x box jump
20 x wallball
10 x hspu

session 266

strength/skill:
front squat 6 x 2

WOD: AMRAP 8min

5 x hang squat snatch (40/30)
10 x bar facing burpees
15 x toes to bar

session 267

strength/skill:
pull up 4 x max effort

WOD: 4 rounds

AMRAP 4 min
4 x squat clean (50/35)
6 x O/H squat
4 x shoulder to overhead
6 x jumping lunge (each leg)
rest 90 sec

session 268

strength/skill:
4 x complex- strict press/push presh/push jerk

WOD: with 25 min cap
run 1.6 km

then

get as far through open workout 14.5 as possible

21/18/15/12/9/6/3
thrusters
bar over burpees

session 269

strength/skill:
handstand prac:
3x12 hspu if possible

WOD: for time

50 x pull ups
25 x lunges (each leg)
40 x hspu
20 x lunges
30 x toes 2 bar
15 x lunges
20 x box jumps
10 x lunges
10 x muscle ups
5 x lunges

session 270

strength/skill:
deadlift 5 x 5

WOD: AMRAP - 10 min
wallball x 12
hollow rock x 10
ring row x 8
100m sprint

session 271

strength/skill:
back squat find 5 rm
then
EMOM- 6 min. 3 back squats @ 5RM weight

WOD: Buy in- 10 burpees
3 Rounds of
double under x 40 (120 singles)
sit up x 30
kb swing x 20 (20/16)
Buy out- 20 burpees

session 272

strength/skill:
4 x complex of power clean/power clean/full clean/hang power clean

WOD: open WOD 14.2

from 0:00-3:00
2 rounds of
10x O/H squat (40/30)
10 x chest to bar pull up

from 3:00-6:00
2 rounds
12 x O/H squat
12 x C2B

from 6:00-9:00
2 rounds
14 x O/H squat
14 x C2B

continue this sequence until allocated reps are not completed in allotted time

session 273

strength/skill:
4 x press complex - strict press x 6/ push press x 2

WOD: AMRAP 15 min

deadlift x 4 (130/90)
push up x 8
squat x 16
run 200m

session 274

strength/skill:

ring dips 4 x 10 (weighted if possible)

WOD: 30 RFT
squat clean x 1 (70/50)
burpee x 3

session 275

strength/skill:
10 min running clock
5 x pull ups every 30 seconds

WOD: AMRAP- 20 min
box jump x 12
front rack lunge x 12 (6 each leg) 50/35
toes to bar x 12

session 276

strength/skill:
pull up 4 x10 (weighted if possible)

WOD: 8 x 90 sec rounds
thruster x 5 (40/30)
50m sprint
max effort bar over burpees
rest 90 secs

session 277
strength/skill:
deadlift 6 x 4

WOD: for time

100 x double under
90 x air squat
80 x push up
70 x box jump
60 x wall ball
50 x pull up

40 x lunges (each leg)
30 x power clean (40/30)
20 x shoulder to over head
10 x deadlift

session 278

strength/skill:
power snatch - work up to a heavy double

WOD: for time
run 1.6km
hang power snatch x 15 (30/20)
power snatch x 10 (40/25)
full snatch x 5 (50/30)
run 1.6km

session 279

strength/skill:
front squat- 10/8/5/5/5/2/2

EMOM- 7 min
jumping back squat x 10

WOD: AMRAP 7 min
sit up x 10
kb snatch x 12 (6 each arm 20/12)
hollow rock x 10
kb clean+press x 12 (6 each arm)

session 280

strength/skill:
find 1rm pull up

WOD: 5 RFT
push press x 10 (50/35)
200m rum

session: 281

strength/skill:

EMOM: 8 min
hang power clean x 3
burpee x 3

WOD: ascending ladder - 12 min
1 x cluster (60/40)
1 x wallball
1 x shuttle run (door to driveway)

2 x cluster
2x wallball
2x shuttle run
etc…..

session 281

strength/skill:
rope climbs (bring long socks!)

hollow holds 5 x 30 sec

WOD: AMRAP 10 min
sit up x 15
kb swing x 15
jumping lunge x 15 (each leg)

session 282

strength/skill:
thruster 5 x 3

WOD: AMRAP 15 min
5 x power clean (70/50)
10 x toes to bar
15 x wall balls

session 283

strength/skill:
overhead squat 5 x 5

WOD: 5 rounds for time
60 x double unders
10 x sumo high pulls (40/30)
10 bar over burpees
1 min rest

session 284

strength/skill:

EMOM: 12 min
even- TnG squat clean x 3 AHAP
odd- 30 second max effort push ups

WOD: AMRAP- 4 min
toes to bar x 7
deadlift x 7 (100/70)

rest 2 min

AMRAP- 4min
100 m sprint
pull up x 7

rest 2 min

AMRAP 5 min
air squat x 14
hang power clean x 7 (50/35)

session 285

strength/skill:

hang power snatch 5 x 3

WOD: for time

15/12/9
thrusters (30/20)
pull ups

rest 2 min

12/9/6
thrusters
pull ups

rest 2 min

9/6/3
thrusters
pull ups

session 286

strength/skill:
muscle up 3 x 5-10

WOD: for time
med ball clean x 30
sit up x 30
med ball clean x 30
push up x 30
med ball clean x 30
ring dips x 30
med ball clean x 30

session 287

strength/skill:
pull ups

WOD: AMRAP 5 min
deadlift x 10 (60/40)
walking lunge x 20

rest 3 min

AMRAP 5 min
shoulder to over head x 7 (30/20)
slam ball x 7 (35/20)

session 288

strength/skill:
back squat 5 x 10

WOD: 4 rounds for time

200m run with med ball
100m run without med ball
20 x lateral jumps over med ball
5 x muscle ups

session 289

strength/skill:
find heaviest complex of- push press/push press/push jerk
(20 min)

AMRAP 15 min
kb swing x 40 (20/12)
c+j x 30 (50/35)
box jump x 20

session 290

strength/skill:
deadlift 6 x 2

WOD:
tabata- push up
rest 1 min
tabata- squat
rest 1 min
tabata- hollow rock

session 291

strength/skill:
EMOM-10 min
even- strict pull up x 10
odd- wall walk x 5

WOD: 12 min clock
4 min amrap of wall ball
4 min amrap of Full clean and jerk (60/40)
4 min amrap bar over burpees

session 292

monster mash courtesy of CrossFit Linchpin

3 rounds for time:
squat clean x 9 (50/35)
push press x 15

rest 5 min

E2MO2M -20 min
20 air squat
100 m sprint

rest 5 min

5 rounds for time
strict ring dips x 12 (box dips)
strict pull ups x 12 (ring rows)

session 293

strength/skill:
bench press 5 x 5

WOD: ascending ladder 2/4/6/8 etc.. 12 min

hollow rock

rope climb x 2 after each round of hollow rock

session 294

open workout 15.1

session 295

strength/skill:
power clean 5/5/3/3/1/1

WOD: AMRAP 9 min
O/H squat x 8 (50/35)
C2B x 12
100m sprint

session 296

strength/skill:
EMOM- 12 min
even- dip x 10
odd- L-sit hold (30 secs)

WOD: 12 min running clock
amrap 3 min- box jumps
amrap 3 min- burpee pull up
amrap 2 min- box jumps
amrap 2 min- burpee pull up
amrap 1 min- box jumps
amrap 1 min- burpee pull up

session 297

strength:
back squat find 3RM

WOD: for time

run 400 m
4 x bear complex (50/35)
run 300 m
3 x bear complex
run 200 m

2x bear complex
run 100m
1 x bear complex

session 298

monster mash!

75 pull ups
75 push ups
75 front squat (30/20)
75 hang power clean
75 push press
75 double under
(25 min cap)

rest 5 min

3 rounds
400 m run
20 box jump
15 kte
3 rope climbs

rest 5 min

20 snatches (75/50)

session 299

strength/skill:
strict press 4 x 8

WOD: 10/8/6/4/2
single arm kb thruster (16/10) each arm
double under (100/80/60 etc...)

session 300

WOD: murph

1.6 km run
100 pull up
200 push up
300 squats
1.6 km run
divide pull up, push ups and squats as needed.

session 301

strength/skill:
3 x 3 pause snatch (pause at knee, pause in squat)

WOD: 5 rounds for time
5 x front squat (80/50)
20 x wallball

session 302

strength/skill:
bench press 6 x 3

WOD: AMRAP- 12 min

push press x 8 (50/35)
bar over burpee x 10
KB swing x 12 (20/16)

session 303

Friday monster mash!

running clock

from 0:00 - 15:00
3 rounds
12 thrusters (60/40)
6 muscle ups (scaled option- ring dips)

from 15:00-30:00
3 rounds
12 burpee box jumps
6 squat clean (90/60)

from 30:00
3 rounds
12 overhead squats
6 bar muscle ups (scaled option - c2b or jumping c2b)

session 304
strength/skill:
deadlift - 4 x 8

WOD: emom
14 wall ball
16 wall ball
18 wallball
ect....
until reps cant be completed

session 305
open WOD 15.3

session 306

strength/skill:
squat clean- 5/5/3/3/1/1

WOD:
3 rounds for total reps
1 min - thrusters (40/30)
1 min - box jumps
1 min - muscle ups
1 min - sit ups

session 307

strength/skill:
emom 12 min
even- push press x 4
odd- 30 sec hollow hold

WOD: open wod 13.1

17 min amrap
40 burpees
30 snatch (30/20)
30 burpees
30 snatch (60/35)
20 burpees
30 snatch (75/45)
10 burpees
amrap snatch (95/54)

session 308

strength/skill:
deadlift: find close to 3RM
EMOM- 7 min
4 x deadlift @80% of triple (fastest reps possible that form allows)

WOD: 5 x 3 min amraps

hspu x 8
jumping lunges x 16 (8 each leg)
100 sprint

rest 1 min

session 309

moster mash!

5 RFT (15 min cap)
2 x rope climb
6 x power clean (80/50)
12 x ring dips

3 RFT (15 min cap)
400 m run
20 x power snatch (40/30)

2 RFT (15 min cap)
20 x deadlift (70/50)
15 x front squat
15 x S2O
200m run

session 310

strength/skill:
front rack lunges 4 x 12 meters

WOD:

18 x plate thrusters (20/10)
200 m run
50 x double unders
15 x plate thrusters
200 m run
50 x double unders
12 x plate thrusters
200 m run
50 x double unders

session 311
open wod 15.4

session 312
strength/skill:
front squat- 5 x 3
paused front squat 3 x 5 @ 70% of above (3 sec pause at bottom)

WOD: for time
row 500m
20 air squat
row 500m

session 313

strength/skill
hang power clean 3/3/3/3

WOD:21/15/9
toes to bar
power clean (60/40)

session 314

strength/skill:
pull up

WOD:
800 m run
burpee box jump x 30
kb swing x 30
box jump x 20
push up x 20
burpee box jump x 10
muscle up x 10
800 m run

session 315

monster mash!

session 316

strength/skill:
bench press 20/20/10/10

WOD: 5 rounds for time
wallball x 15
push up x 10
sit up x 15

session 316

open wod 15.5

session 317

strength/skill:
ring dips 5 x 10

WOD: 21/15/9
deadlift (100/70)
bar facing burpee

session 318

strength skill:
split jerk 5 x 1

WOD:
50 x back squat (40/30)
50 x pull up
50 x front squat
50 x push up

session 319

strength/skill:
for 6 min- every 30 sec: cluster
rest 1 min
emom- 6 min: clean and jerk x 2
rest 1 min
emom- 6 min: squat clean
(aim is to increase load at each rest)

WOD: For time
1.6 km run

session 320

strength/skill:
O/H squat - 6 x 2

WOD: AMRAP 8 min
push press x 8 (50/35)
kb sumo high pull x 12 (20/16)

session 320

Strength/skill:
muscle up prac

WOD: 15 min amrap

25 bar over burpees
21 clusters (30/20)
25 BOB
15 clusters (40/30)
25 BOB
9 clusters (50/35)
25 BOB
AMRAP clusters (60/40)

session 321
strength/skill:
10 min clock- 5 x strict pull up every 30 secs

WOD: 10 rounds
 1 min amrap
8 x deadlift (60/40)
6 x hang power clean
4 x front squat
2 x push jerk
max effort wallballs in remaining
 1 min rest

score is wallballs

session 322

monster mash!

session 323

strength/skill:
front squat- 4 x 12

WOD: 10 -1
box step overs with KB (16/12)
push up

13/4/15
strength/skill:
bench press- 5 x 3

WOD: 3 rounds @ 100%
200 m sprint
10 x kb swing (20/16)
10 x burpee
10 x kb swing
10 x burpee
10 x kb swing
200 m sprint
rest 5 min

session 324

Strength/skill:
deadlift- find 3rm

WOD:
30 x thruster (30/20)
20 x pull up
10 x burpee
rest 90 sec

20 x thruster (40/30)
15 x c2b pull up
10 x burpee
rest 90 sec

10 x thruster (50/35)

10 x burpee pull up

session 325

strength/skill: emom- 10 min
hang power clean x 5

WOD: AMRAP 11 min
11 x box jumps
11 x hang power clean (40/30)

session 326

strength/skill:
push press 5/3/3/1/1/1

WOD: 5 rounds for time

20 x O/H squat (30/20)
50 x double under

session 327

moster mash

session 328

strength/skill:
front rack lunges 5 x 12m

WOD: 30/20/10
calories on rower
wallballs

session 329

strength/skill:

snatch 3/3/2/2/1/1

WOD: AMRAP 8 min
20 x jumping lunge
10 x burpee

sessio 330

strength/skill:
ring row 4 x 10 (3 sec pause at top)

WOD: 3 rounds for time
14 x toes to bar
7 x push press (50/35)

rest 5 min

15/12/9
ring dips
100m with plate overhead (20/10)

session 331

strength/skill:
muscle up

WOD: ascending ladder 12 min

box jump
pull up

1,1,
2,2,
3,3, etc….

rest 5 min

500m row

session 332

strength/skill:
bench press- 3 x 8

WOD: 2 rounds for time
400 m run
50 x double under
50 x thruster (20/15)
50 x push up
5 x muscle up

session 323
monster mash

session 324

anzac day hero wod

session 325

strength/skill:
thruster -5/5/3/3/1/1

WOD: death by thruster (40/30)
0-1 min - 1 thruster
1-2 min - 2 thrusters
2-3 min - 3 thrusters
continue this pattern until thrusters can't be completed

session 326

strength/skill:
pull up 4 x max effort

WOD: 10-1
plyo push up (6'/3')
kb snatch (20/12) each arm

session 327

strength/skill:
front squat find 1rm

WOD: 6 min clock
1 min amrap -power clean (60/40)
1 min amrap - wall ball
1 min amrap - hollow rock
1 min amrap - toes to bar
1 min amrap - lateral jumps over bar
1 min amrap - bar over burpees
rest 3 min
repeat

session 328

strength/skill:
accumulate 3 min in hanging L-sit

EMOM- 8 min
cluster/push press/ split jerk

WOD:
200 skips
400m row
800m run
200 skips

session   329

monster mash

session 330
strength/skil:
emom - 12 min
odd- headstand hold
even - hollow rock

WOD: chelsea
EMOM 30 min
5 x pull up
10 x push up
15 x squat

session 331

strength/skill:
find 1 rm strict press
rest 4 min
then emom 5 min- 2 reps @ 90% of 1rm

WOD: for time
jumping lunge x 20
hang power snatch x 10 (30/20)
wallball x 20
hang power snatch x 10
wallball x 30
hang power snatch x 10
wallball x 40
jumping lunge x 20

session   332

strength/skill:
deadlift- 5 x 3

WOD: 15 min ascending ladder
squat clean (60/40)
bar over burpee
2,4,6,8,10 etc…

session 333

strength/skill:
O/H squat- 3 x 3

WOD: 5 rounds for time
20 x pull up
20 x push up
400 m run

session 334
strength/skill:

bench press- 5 x 2

WOD: 15/12/9/6
burpee box jump
ring dip
TTB

session 335
mosnter mash

session 336

strength/skill:
back squat 3 x10

WOD- 12 min amrap 'wod for nepal'
8x thruster (60/40)
8 x hang power clean
4 x muscle up
8 x front rack lunges

scaled version
8 x S2O (40/30)
8 x hang power clean
4 x burpee
8 x front rack lunge

session 337

strength/skill:
power clean 6 x 2

WOD: for time
squat x 80
push jerk x 20 (50/35)
squat x 60
push jerk x 15
squat x 40
push jerk x 10
squat x 20

push jerk x 5

session 338

strength/skill:
handstand push up 4 x 5-10 (deficit if possible)

WOD: fran

21/15/9
thrusters (40/30)
pull ups

session 339

strength/skill:
ring dips 5 x 3-5 (weighted)

WOD:
7 rounds
100 m shuttle run
30 L-sit hold
10 x burpee to target

rest 1 min

session 340

strength/skill:
pendlay row 5 x 5

WOD:
 AMRAP - 4 min
wallball x 8
sumo high pull x 8 (40/30)
rest 1 min

AMRAP- 3 min
wallball x 6
sumo high pull x 6

rest 1 min

AMRAP - 2 min
wallball x 4
sumo high pull x 4
rest 30 sec

AMRAP - 1 min
wallball x 2
sumo high pull x 2

session   341
monster mash

session 342

strength/skill:
push press 5 x 3

WOD:
EMOM
1- 1 x burpee
2- 4 x jumping lunge
3- 3 x burpee
4- 8 x jumping lunge
5- 5 x burpee
6- 12 x jumping lunge
7- 7 x burpee
8- 16 x jumping lunge
continue pattern until failure

session   343

strength/skill:
EMOM 7 min-
power clean, squat clean, hang squat clean

EMOM 7 min-
squat clean, hang squat clean

EMOM 7 min-
hang squat clean

WOD: tabata
alternating- push up/kb swing (20/16)
rest 1 min
alternating- sit ups/planking (plank as rest)

session 343

strength/skill: back squat
5 x 3 (33X2 tempo)

WOD: AMRAP 15 min
200 m run
10 x wallballs
5 x thruster (60/40)

session 344

strength/skill:
hang power snatch - 6 x 2

WOD:
21 x deadlift (100/70)
21 x pull up
10 x burpee box jump
15 x deadlift
15 x pull up
10 x burpee box jump
9 x deadlift
9 x pull up
10 x burpee box jump

6pm class
warm up- dynamic
then
squat tech
then
wall ball teams- first to get through 5 rounds
repeat a few times

WOD 1
10-1
plate thruster
push up
jump lunge

WOD 2
death by burpee

session 345

strength/skill:
split jerk - 5 x 1

WOD: for time
1.5k row
straight into 3 min amrap
burpee broad jump

session 346
monstermash

session 347

strength/skill:
bench press 4 x 8

WOD: 4 rounds 1 min max effort at each station
rowing (calories)
box jump
clean and jerk (50/35)
deadball to shoulder (35/20)
deficit push ups (6"/3")

session 348

strength/skill:
O/H squat - 5 x 5

WOD: ascending ladder - 12 min (3,6,9,etc..)
squat snatch (30/20)
pull up

session 349

strength/skill:
ring dips 5 x 5 (pause at bottom range for 5 sec)

WOD: for time
buy in/out: double unders- 50/100

Racked KB lunges x 60 (30 each leg) (20/16)
run 400m with wall ball
box step overs with wall ball x 30
run 400m with wall ball
single KB o/h squat x 20 (10 each arm)

session 350

strength/skill:
deadlift 5 x 5

WOD: for time
(every 2 min perform 15 air squats)
TTB x 75
push up x 75
sit up x 50
wallball x 50
KB sumo high pull x 25 (20/16)
burpee x 25

session 351

strength/skill:
strict press- 5 x 5

WOD: 3 rounds for time
power clean x 15 (40/30)
thruster x 10
200m run

session 352
monster mash

session 353

strength/skill:
ring push ups - 5 x 12

WOD: 5 rounds
30 sec L-sit hold (hanging from bar)
box jump x 20
hollow rock x 20

rest

tabata- row

session 354

strength/skill:
20 min to find heaviest complex of- squat clean/hang power clean/split jerk

WOD: for time

30 burpee muscle ups
or
30 burpee pull ups straight into 30 dips

session 355
strength/skill:
bench press - find 1RM

WOD:- Dianne
21/15/9
deadlift (100/70)
HSPU

session 356

strength/skill: muscle ups

WOD: kalsu
100 x thruster (60/40)
5 burpees emom

session 357

strength/skill:
pull up 5 x 15

WOD: 5 RFT
O/H lunge x 12 (6 each leg, 50/35)
box jump x 12
200 m run

session 358
monster mash

session   359

strength/skill:
back squat 3 x 12

WOD:
 3 rounds
row 300m
run 200m

session 360
strength/skill:
deadlift 3 x 8

WOD:
For time:
   ◦   30 Bear Complexes 50/35

For this workout a "bear complex" will consist of:
   ◦   Power clean

- Front squat
- Push press or Push jerk
- Back squat
- Push press or Push Jerk

*Note, you may combine the 1st 3 parts into a "squat clean thruster"
*You can "rest" in the hang, front rack, overhead, or back rack

*IF YOU DROP THE BAR you must perform 3 burpees, 4 toes to bar, and 5 wall ball shots 20/14 before picking up the barbell again

session 361

strength/skill:
hang power clean 5 x 3

WOD: 3 x 3min AMRAP
hang power clean x 5 (60/40)
lateral bar jumps x 30
rest 2 min

session 362

strength/skill:
chest to bar pull up - 4 x 10

WOD:AMRAP 12 min
40m walking lunge with plate overhead (15/10)
30 x wallball
25 x kb swing (20/16)
20 x box jump
15 x snatch (50/30)
amrap rope climb in remainder time

session 363

monster mash

session 364

eva or kelly

session 365
strength/skill:
EMOM 10min: 7 x hspu

WOD: for time
thruster x 40 (30/20)
sit up x 40
thruster x 25 (40/30)
sit up x 40
thruster x 15 (50/35)
sit up x 40
thruster x 10 (60/40)
sit up x 40
thruster x 5 (70/45)

session 366

strength/skill:
5 x complex of - 2 x strict press/3 x push press/ 4 x push jerk

WOD: for time
21/15/9
deadlift (125/90)
burpee boxjump

session 367

strength/skill:
find 1rm squat clean

WOD: for time
40 x muscle up
EMOM- 2 x squat clean (60/40)

session 368

strength/skill:
bench press 5 x 5

WOD: AMRAP 15 min
sumo high pull x 5 (60/40)
TTB x 10
double under x 30

session 369
monster mash

session 370

front rack lunges 5 x 10m

WOD: barbara

session 371
strength/skill:
back squat 5/5/3/3/3

WOD: amrap 8 min
wallball x 8
broad jump x 20m

session 372

Skill: rope climb tech

WOD: 7 rounds
1 x rope climb
30 x kb swing (20/16)
1 x rope climb
30 x kb snatch (15 Each arm)

session   373

strength/skill:
hang squat snatch - 2/2/1/1/1/1

WOD: for time
buy in - row 750 m
then
jump lunge x 80
push up x 60
sit up x 40
burpee x 20
sit up x 40
push up x 60
jump lunge x 80

session 374

strength/skill:
1RM deadlift

WOD: 3 rounds

amrap 4 min
O/H squat x 6 (50/35)
hang power clean x 8
burpee x 6

rest 2 min

session 375
monster mash

session 376

strength/skill:
thruster - 5/5/3/3/3

WOD:

light Fran 15/12/6- thrusters (30/20)/ pull ups
400 m run
light Fran
400 m run

session   377

strengh/skill:
front squat 6 x 3

WOD: AMRAP 6 min
med ball clean x 8
burpee x 10

session 378

strength/skill:
pull up 5 x 5 (weighted)

WOD: 5 rounds
2 min running clock

deadlift x 4 (140/90)
lateral jumps over bar x 12
remainder time amrap of HR push ups
rest 2 min

session 379

strength/skill:
EMOM- 12 min
power clean/hang squat clean/ push press/ split jerk

WOD:
400m run

5 min rest

Half Cindy - 10 min amrap
5 x pull up
10 x push up
15 x squat

session 380

strength/skill:
weighted muscle up - 5 x 2

WOD:
hspu x 30
double under x 100
hspu x 25
double under x 100
hspu x 20
double under x 100
hspu x 15
double under x 100
hspu x 10
double under x 100
hspu x 5
double under x 100

session 381

monstermash

session 382

strength/skill:
bench press 5 x 4

WOD: tabata row

then 2 x

all exercises in same tabata
push press (30/20)
box jump
burpee
wallball
(8 rounds in a tabata means each exercise will be performed twice, rest 2 min
between tabatas)

session 383
strength/skill:
pistol squats

WOD: Grace

30 clean and jerks (60/40)

session 384

strength/skill:
paused O/H squats 5 x 3 (33X0)

WOD: 50/40/30/20/10
Pull ups
HR push ups
(1 x power clean every 2min 80/55)

session 385

strength/skill:
halted clean deadlift - 5 x 5

WOD:
WOD: for time
21/15/9
ring dips
front squat (40/30)

rest 3 min

18/15/12
hang power clean (50/35)
air squat

session 386

strength/skill:
power clean 3 x 2
hang power clean 3 x 1

WOD: AMRAP 8 min
cluster x 5 (60/40)
wallball x 10

session 387

strength/skill:
split jerk 7 x 1

WOD: 5 x 250m row

session 388

strength/skill:
front lever

WOD:
8 x bar over burpee
5 x clean (60/40)

rest 1 min

8 x BOB
4 x clean (70/45)

rest 1 min

8 x BOB
3 x clean (80/50)

rest 1 min

8 x BOB
2 x clean (90/55)

rest 1 min

8 x BOB
1 x clean (100/60)

session 388

strength/skill:
strict press - 4 x 6

WOD: AMRAP 20 min

wallball x 30
muscle up x 5
hang power snatch x 20 (30/20)
muscle up x 5

session 389
monster mash

session   390

strength/skill:
front lunges 4 x 20m

WOD: 8 rounds
1 min clock
deadlift x 3 (110/80)
50m sprint
amrap burpees in remainder time
rest 2 min

session 391

strength/skill:
back squat 3/3/3/2/2/2

WOD: for time
21/15/9
dips
push ups

session 392

strength/skill:
pull up - 5 x 3 weighted

WOD: 9/6/3
O/H squat (60/40)
strict C2B pull up

rest 3 min

12/9/6

O/H squat (50/35)
strict pull up

rest 3 min

15/12/9
O/H squat (40/30)
pull up

session 393

srength/skill:
deadlift 3 x 5

WOD:
21/15/9/15/21
push press (50/35)
KTE

session 394
strength/skill:
find heavy a complex of - squat clean/front squat

WOD: AMRAP 10 min
front squat x 7 (70/45)
KB snatch x 7 each arm (20/16)
sit up x 7

24/7/15

monster mash

session 396

strength/skill:
push press 3 x 5.

WOD: angie
100 x pull up
100 x push up
100 x squat

100 x sit up

session 397

strength/skill:
hang power snatch 5 x 2

WOD: AMRAP 12 min
thruster x 8 (50/35)
hang power clean x 6
muscle up x 4

session 398

strength/skill:
bench press 3 x 10

WOD:
100 m O/H lunges with plate (20/15)
90 x KB swing (20/16)
80 x double unders
70 m O/H lunges
60 x KB swing
50 x double under
40 m O/H lunge
30 x KB swing
20 x double under
10 x burpee

session 399

strength/skill:
pig squat for load
20-1 front squat
start with empty bar, each round decreases 1 rep while increasing in weight,
aiming to end close to your current 1RM
rest as needed between sets

session 400

WOD:
400 m run
5 min rest
half cindy 10 min amrap

5 pull up
10 push up
15 squat

session 401

onster mash

session 402

strength/skill:
turkish get up 3 x 3 each arm

WOD:
10-1
clean (50/35)
push press
(1 lap waiters walk (20/16) every 2 min)

session 403
strength/skill:
strict press 5 x 3 (x233 tempo)

WOD: 4 rounds of
30 on 30 off
air squat
box jump
burpee
wallball
score is total reps

session 404

strength/skill:
pull up 4 x max effort

WOD: 4 rounds for time

deadlift x 10 (140/95)
ring dip x 20
TTB x 30

session 405

strength/skill:
emom - 21 min
1- complex- power clean/hang squat clean/split jerk
2- double under x 25 (or 35 sec amrap)
3- push up x 25 (or 35 sec amrap)

WOD: AMRAP 10 min
front lunge x 12 (60/40)
kb thruster x 12 (6 each arm 20/16)

session 406

strength/skill:
bench press 5 x 5

WOD: 5 rounds for time
10 x ground to overhead (40/30)
15 x burpee

session 407
monster mash

session 408

strength/skill:
muscle up

WOD: EMOM - 40 min
1- row 15/12 calories
2- round of cindy
3- run 100m

4- 12 burpees

session 409
strength/skill:
power clean 5 x 2

WOD: amrap 3 min
deadlift x 3 (140/90)
bar over burpee x 3

1 min rest

amrap 3 min
deadlift x 5 (100/70)
BOB x 5

1 min rest
amrap 3 min
BOB

session   410
strength/skill:
5 x 3 weighted dips

WOD:
48/24/12
thrusters (20/15)
wallballs

Session 411
strength/skill:
ghd sit up 3 x10
hip exstension 3 x10

WOD: 7 rounds
7 x weighted pull up (20lb/14lbs)
7 x burpee box ump
7 x hang power clean (70/45)

session 412
strength/skill:
back squat- 6 x 2

WOD: for time
cluster x 50 (50/35)

session 413
monster mash

session 414
strength/skill:
ring push up variations

WOD: partner wod

30 min running clock

partner 1 runs 200m with med ball
partner 2 performs amrap of thrusters   (30/20)

partner 1 skips 150 skips
partner 2 performs amrap of slam ball over shoulder

partner 1 runs 200m with med ball
partner 2 performs amrap of pullups/ring rows

partner 1 skips 150 skips
partner 2 performs amrap of wall balls

go back to start and swap roles

session 415
strength/skill:
push press 3 x 5
push jerk 3 x 2

WOD: 4 rounds for time
med ball clean x 25
muscle up x 5

session 416
strength/skill:
deadlift - 3 reps every 2 min for 14 min AHAP

WOD:
amrap - 20 min
toes to ring x 100
squat x 50
bear complex x 25 (40/30)
(*bear complex- power clean/front squat/push press/back squat /push press)

session 417
strength/skill: 5 x complex power snatch/ hang squat snatch

WOD: for time
100 box jumps
2 x power cleans every 90secs (80/55)

session 418
strength/skill:
emom- 21min
1- 10 x strict pull up
2- 10 x hspu (or 30 sec hs hold)
3- 30 sec l-sit

WOD: AMRAP- 10 min
box step up with kb x 8 (20/16) each leg
HR push up x 10

sesssion 419
monster mash

session 420

strength/skill:
bench press - 3 x 10

WOD: deck of cards fran
in two teams for 25 min

black card - thrusters (value on card determines the number of reps)
red card - pull ups
picture card - burpees x 10
joker - 400 m run

session 421
strength/skill:
clean pull + clean - 2+1 x 4
halting segment clean 3 x 3 @ 80-90% of clean 1rm

WOD:
tabata sit up
1 min rest
tabata jump lunge
1 min rest
tabata burpee broad jump
1 min rest
tabata jump lunge

session 422
strength/skill:
C2B - 4 x 10

WOD: 0-3min
cluster x 6 (50/35)
TTB x 6

3-6min
cluster x 8
TTB x 8

6-9 min
cluster x 10
TTB x 10

9-12min
cluster x 12
TTB x 12

12-15min
cluster x 14
TTB x 14

etc.... until failure to complete reps in round

session 423
strength/skill:
front rack lunges 5 x 12 meters

WOD:
400m run
60 x air squat
30 x push up
10 x hang power snatch (40/30)
30 x push up
60 x air squat
400 m run

session 424

strength/skill:
strict press x3 /push press x 2 - x 5

WOD: 3 rounds
12 x thruster (50/35)
9 x hang power clean
6 x bar facing burpee
3 x rope climb

session 425
monster mash

session 426

strength/skill:
back squat 3 x 10

WOD: in two teams
complete 3k row
400 x walking lunges
100 x ghd sit ups

session 427

strength/skill:
clean and jerk- 5 x 2

WOD: 3/6/9/12/15
muscle up
O/H squat (60/40)

session 428

strength/skill:
L-sit 3 x max effort
hand stand 3 x max effort

WOD: 2 rounds for time
100 m walking lunge
100 m walk with 2 plates in pinch grip (15/10)
100 m broad jump
100 hollow rocks

session 429
strength/skill:
rope climb practice

WOD: 6 rounds for time
3 x snatch (60/40)
2 x rounds of cindy
1 x rope climb

session 430

strength/skill:
push jerk 5 x 2

WOD: "DT"
5 rounds for time
12 x deadlift (70/50)
9 x hang power clean
6 x push jerk

session 431

Monster mash

session 432

strength/skill:
O/H walking lunge 3 x 12m

WOD: 5 rounds for time
15 x KB swing (32/24)
15 x burpee

session 433

WOD:
4 x 400m run (rest 2 min between efforts)
3 x 300m row rest as needed

no one like these sessions, but if your serious, they are necessary.

session 434

strength/skill:
front squat 7 x 2

WOD: AMRAP 6 min
burpee x 5
squat clean x 2 (60/40)

session 435

strength/skill:
pull up 5 x 5 weighted

WOD: 5 rounds
hang power snatch x 7 (40/30)
wall ball x 9
push up x 11

session 436

strength/skill:
find 1 RM ring dip (or 4 x 10 assisted)

WOD: 4 rounds
deadlift x 10 (125/80)
box jump x 20
200m sprint
rest 2 min between rounds

session 437

monster mash
4-5-6-7-8 reps for time of:
Bar Muscle-ups
Wall Balls 20/14 (4x reps)

AMRAP 9 minutes of:
9 Calories Rowing
6 Burpees over rower
3 Clean & Jerks 185/125

4 Rounds for time of:
60 double-unders
15 Kettle Bell Swings 53/35
15 Hollow Rocks
Rest 5 minutes between workouts.

session 438
partner wod:
complete as pairs (one working, one resting)
100 x thrusters (40/30)
90 x box jumps
80 x sit ups
70 x jumping lunges
60 x goblet squat (20/16)
50 x push ups
40 x burpees
30 x wall balls
20 x pull ups
10 x 100m sprints

session 439

strength/skill:
O/H squat- 5 x 5

WOD: Heavy fran
21/15/9
thrusters (50/35)
pull ups (20lbs/14lbs)

session 440
strength/skill:
bench press- 10/8/6/4/6/8/10

WOD: AMRAP 10 min
burpee box jump x 12
sit up x 20

session 441
strength/skill:
deadlift 6 x 2

WOD:
ascending ladder 8 min
HR push up
front squat (50/35)
2/4/6/8/10 etc.....

session 442

strength/skill:
EMOM 6 min
30 sec hand stand hold

EMOM 12 min
even- hollow rock x 12
odd- 30 sec l-sit hold

WOD: in 2 teams row as far as possible in 20 min swapping every 1 min.
also teams must accumulate 150 sit ups (only 1 person at a time doing sit ups)

session 443
strength/skill:
front squat- 4 x 4
paused front squat 3 x 2 (3 sec pause)

WOD: AMRAP 9 min
hang power clean x 3 (60/40)
2 rounds of cindy
(* cindy- 5 x pull up/ 10x push up/ 15 x squat)

session 444
monster mash

session 445
strength/skill:
pull up 5 x 15 (beginners- 4 x 5-10)

WOD: 8 x 2 min rounds
200m run
8 x wallball
8 x jumping lunge each leg
amrap of bupree in remainder

90 sec rest

session 446
strength/skill:
strict press- 5 x 5
push press- 5 x 1

WOD:AMRAP - 4 min
box jump x 6
burpee pull up x 6
rest 90 sec

AMRAP - 3 min
box jump x 4
burpee pull up x 4

rest 90sec

AMRAP -2 min
burpee pull up

session 447
strength/skill:
front rack lunge 5 x 20m

WOD: 3 rounds for time
21 x toes to bar
15 x HR push up
9 x sumo high pull (60/40)

session 448
strength/skill:
rope climb - 8 ascents (rest as needed)

WOD: for time
50 x ghd sit up
50 x kb swing (20/16)
50 x dips
50 x push press (40/30) no jerks!
50 x O/H squat (40/30)
50 x hang power clean (40/30)

session 449
strength/skill:
squat clean - 3/2/2/1/1//2/2/3

WOD: AMRAP 6 min
jumping lunge with wall ball over head x 10 (5 EL)
burpee x 10

session 450
monster mash

session 451
WODS:

AMRAP- 4 min
rowing (calories)
rest 2 min

AMRAP- 4 min
burpee to target (6")
rest 2 min

AMRAP - 4 min
wallball
rest 2 min

AMRAP - 4 min
50m shuttle run
rest 2 min

AMRAP- 4 min
plate thruster (20/15)
rest 2 min

AMRAP- 4min
box jump

session 452
strength/skill:
back squat- 10/5/3/2/1/1/2/3/5/10

WOD:AMRAP 5 min
thruster x 12 (40/30)
kb swing x 12 (20/16)

session 453
strength/skill:
bench press- 5 x 2 (2 sec pause at chest)

WOD: 3 rounds for time
300m shuttle run (100m x 3)
kb sumo high pull x 15 (32/24)

session 454
strength/skill:

5 sets of
30 sec L-sit straight into 20 hollow rocks
rest 1 min

WOD: 2 rounds
25 x front squat (60/40)
25 x box jump
12 x push press
25 x box jump
25 x bar facing burpee

session 455
strength/skill:
pull up 4 x 4 weighted

WOD: 25 rounds for time
2 x muscle up
1 x deadlift (150/105)

session 456
monster mash

session 457
strength/skill:
front squat 4 x 12

WOD: 4 rounds for time
double under x 50
wallball x 20

session 458
strength/skill:
find 1rm cluster

WOD: 3 rounds for time
200m run
5 x cluster @ 80%

rest 5 min

12/9/6

200m run
cluster @ 50%

session 459
strength/skill:
weighted dips - 5/3/2/3/5

WOD: AMRAP 20 min
box jump x 15
pull up x 10
push up x 15
sumo high pull x 10 (50/35)

session 460

strength/skill:
power clean 3 x 2
hang power clean 2 x 2

WOD:
6 x 45 sec row for calories

session   461

strength/skill:
split jerk - 4 x 2

WOD: 4 rounds for time
21 x O/H squat (50/35)
15 x bar facing burpees
9 x thrusters

session 462
monster mash

session 463
strength/skill:
ring rows - 5 x 10

WOD:

0-3 min:
box jump x 10
wall ball x 10

3-6 min:
box jump x 12
wallball x 12

6-9 min:
box jump x 14
wallball x 14

continue this pattern until failure to complete reps in time slot

session 464

strength/skill:
hang power snatch 5 x 2

WOD: 2 rounds for time
push up x 50
deadlift x 25 (50/35)
sit up x 50
push press x 25 (50/35)
jumping lunge x 50

session 465
strength/skill:
EMOM - 14 min
even- 10 x strict pull up
odd- 15 x KB swing AHAP

WOD: for time
10 thrusters (60/40)
20 clean and jerks
10 thrusters

session 466
Strength/skill:
back squat 6 x 2

WOD: amrap- 6 min
burpee x 7
front rack lunge x 7 each leg (40/30)

session 467
strength/skill:
bench press - 5 x 5

WOD:
3 rounds for time
400m run
5 x muscle up
30 x push up
5 x burpee

session 468

monster mash
"Ascending ""Elizabeth"
9-15-21 reps for time of:
Squat Clean 135/95
Ring dips

4 Rounds for time of:
12 Toes to bar
12 Push Jerks 135/95
12 Box Jumps 24""/20""

"SQT"
3 Rounds for time of:
10 Ground to Overhead 95/65
200yd Shuttle Run (50yd x 4)

session 469

strength/skill:
strict press 3 x 8
push press 3 x 5

WOD: 12 min running clock

75 partner sit ups (arms interlocked)
100 partner push ups (1 per person until 100 reached)

in remanding time
AMRAP of KB goblet squats (1 for 1) every time a KB is put down = 10
burpees

session 470

strength/skill:
find heavy complex of
muscle clean/hang power clean/squat clean

WOD: 15 min AMRAP
21 x deadlift (100/70)
21 x HSPU
15 x deadlift
15 x HSPU
9 x dealift
9 x HSPU
100 x wallballs

session 471

strength/skill:
push press 5 x 3

WOD:
buy in - 1.6 km run

then
3 Rounds
8 x hang power snatch (40/30)
12 x TTB

Buy out - 100 x double unders

session 472

strength/skill:
muscle up progressions

WOD: for time
20 x muscle ups
30 x ring dips

40 x push ups
50 x shoulder to overhead (30/20)
60 x box jumps

(*2 x KB snatch each arm every 2 min 32/20)

session 473

strength/skill:
deadlift 5 x 3

WOD: amrap - 7 min
12 x wallball
6 x power clean (70/50)

session 474
monster mash

session 475

strength/skill:
front rack lunges
5 x 12m

WOD: AMRAP 5 min
10 x push up
10 x KB sumo high pull

rest 90 sec

AMRAP 4 min
8 x sit up
8 x wallball

rest 90 sec

AMRAP - 3 min
6 x ring row
1 x lap of broad jumps

rest 90 sec

AMRAP- 2 min
100 m sprint
10 x box step ups (5 each leg 24/20)

rest 90 sec

AMRAP 1 min
burpees

session 476

strength/skill:
front squat 6 x 2

WOD: partner AMRAP - 8 min

partner 1 - hold bar over head (50/35)
partner 2 - TTB x 8
once TTB are completed
partner 2 - hang off bar
partner 1 - S2O x 8

then swap

reps don't count if partner is not holding position

session 477

strength/skill:
bench press - 3 x 10

WOD: 5 RFT
rope climb x 2
wallball x 20
400m run

session 478

strength/skill:
o/h squat - 5 x 3

WOD: AMRAP 12 min
hspu x 8
bear complex x 3 (60/40)

*bear complex- power clean/front squat/ push press/ back squat/push press.

session 479

strength/skill:
find 1rm clean and jerk

WOD: 10-1
clean and jerk (60/40)
pull up

session 480

monster mash

session 481

WOD:
In 2 teams, row 12km for time

session 482

strength/skill:
O/H lunges - 5 x 12m

WOD: for time
100 burpee broad jumps

session 483

strength/skill:
snatch - 3/3/2/2/1/1

WOD: 3 rounds for time
21 x burpee
15 x air squat
9 x hang power snatch (50/35)

session 484

strength/skill:
EMOM - 21 min
1-7min - clean/ hang clean/ clean
7-14min - 2 x clean with 3 sec pause in hole
14-21min - clean

(aim to increase weight each section)

WOD: AMRAP 6 min
8 x pull up
12 x push up

session 485
monster mash
22-16-10 reps for time of:
Chest-to-bar Pull-ups
Overhead Squats 50/30

4 Rounds for time of:
400m run
10 Deadlifts 140/90
20 Wallball Shots 20/14

AMRAP 7 minutes of:
3 Bar Muscle-ups
5 Handstand Push-ups
7 Toes-to-bar

*Rest 5 minutes between workouts.

session 486

strength/skill:
KB strict press 4 x 8
KB push press 3 x 3

WOD: 3 x AMRAP 4 min

air squat x 20
KB sumo high pull x 10 (20/16)

rest 2 min

session 487

strength/skill:
hang squat clean 6 x 2

WOD: 3 rounds for time
12 x thruster (50/35)
12 x jumping lunge Each leg
12 x push up
12 x hang power clean

session 488

strength/skill:
pull up - 4 x 5

WOD: for time
1.6 km run
30 x S2O (60/40)
800m run
15 x S2O
400m run
7 x S2O
200m run
3 x S2O

session 489

strength/skill:

pistol squats 4 x 10 each leg

WOD: AMRAP 20 min
4 x muscle up
8 x deadlift (140/100)
12 x box jump
16 x push up
20 x air squat

session 490

strength/skill:
bench press 5 x 5

WOD: 15 min running clock
200 x double unders (500 singles)
20 x bar facing burpee
10 x rope climbs
in remaing time amrap of squat snatch (60/40)

session 491
monster mash

session 492

strength/skill:
back squat 4 x 10

WOD: AMRAP - 10 min
200m run
12 x plate thruster (20/15)
push up x 10

rest 5 min

tabata hollow rock

session 493
strength/skill:

muscle up prac

WOD:
15 x clean and jerk (70/45)
200 m run
10 x thruster
400 m run
10 x thruster
200 m run
15 x clean and jerk

session 494

strength/skill:
strict press 5 x 3

WOD: AMRAP 20 min
4 x muscle up
8 x deadlift (140/100)
12 x box jump
16 x push up
20 x air squat

session 495

strength/skill:
back squat - 5 x 5

WOD: 4 rft
front squat x 10 (60/40)
kb swing x 15 (32/24)
TTB x 10

session 496

strength/skill:
EMOM- 15 min
1 - 10 x ring dip
2 - 10 x push up
3 - 7 x kb push press each arm

WOD: AMRAP 12 min
1 x bar muscle up
2 x power clean (80/55)
3 x bar facing burpee

session 497

mash

session   498
strength/skill:
front squat 4 x 10

WOD: for time

100 x double unders
50 x box step up
40 x ring push up
30 x pull up
20 x kb swing (20/16)
30 x pull up
40 x ring push up
50 x box step up
100 x du

session 499

strength/skill:
split jerk 4 x 2

WOD:
400m Run Together
100 See-saw Back Squats (50/35)
75 See-saw Burpees
50 See-saw Pull-ups
25 Wallball
400m Run Together

session 500
strength/skill:
front rack lunge - 3 x 20m

WOD: buy in/out- 50 box step ups with kb overhead (16/12)
10 rounds

10 x hang power clean (40/30)
20 x plate snatch (20/15)
10 x push up

session 501

strength/skill:
deadlift - 4 x 2
then
deadlift - 5 x 3 speed reps @ 70% of above on the minute

WOD: AMRAP - 8 min
wallball x 20
double under x 20

session 502
strength/skill:
overhead squat - 6 x 2

WOD: for time
10 x power snatch (60/40)
20 x bar over burpees
10 x hang squat snatch
20 x bar over burpees
10 x squat snatch

esssion 503

monster mash

session 504

strength/skill:
bench press - 4 x 10

WOD: AMRAP - 18 min

in pairs relay style

5 x wallballs
10 x goblet lunges (20/16)
100m run

session 505

strength/skill:
thruster 5 x 3 (from rack)

WOD: AMRAP 15min
60 x thruster (30/20)
30 x burpee
15 x sumo high pull

session 506

strength/skill:
power snatch - 20 min to find find heavy single
then
EMOM 8 min
2 x power snatch 80% of above

WOD: for time
100 pull ups (10 push ups every 90 secs)

session 507

strentgth/skill:
squat clean - 20 min to find heavy single
then
EMOM 8 min

2 x clean @80% of above

WOD: AMRAP 8 min
200m run
6 x kb snatch each arm (20/16)
3 x kb C+J each arm

session 508

strength/skill:
max effort ring dips x 3

WOD:
50 x wallballs
5 x muscle up
40 x toes to bar
4 muscle up
30 x thrusters (40/30)
3 x muscle up
20 x power clean
2 x muscle up
10 x burpees
1 x muscle up

session 509
mash

session 509

strength/skill:
back squat 3 x 12

WOD: AMRAP 4 min
100m sprint
push up x10

rest 2 min

AMRAP 4 min
wallball x 8
jumping lunge with ball x 8 (4 each leg)

rest 2 min

AMRAP 8 min
100m sprint
push up x 10
wallball x 8
jump lunge with ball x 8

session 510

strength/skill:
push press - 5 x 5

WOD: 3 RFT
10 x clean and jerk (60/40)
30 x wall ball

session 511

strength/skill:
front squat 5 x 3 (5-3-x-0 tempo)

WOD: 5 round for time

9 x deadlift (100/70)
12 x pull up

session 512

strength/skill:

21 min running clock
0-7 EMOM- complex of squat clean/hang power clean/hang squat clean
(AHAP)
7-14 EMOM- TTB x 10, KB swing x 5
14-21 EMOM- same complex as 0-7

WOD: AMRAP 3 min
hang power clean (60/40)

rest 1 min

AMRAP 2 min
hang power snatch (40/30)

session   513

strength/skill:
20 min to find O/H squat 1RM

WOD: For time
100 x double unders
80 x jumping lunges
60 x box jumps
40 x burpees
20 x O/H squat (50/35)

session   514
mash

session 515

strength/skill:
accumulate 3 min in a headstand hold
accumulate 3 min in a L-sit

WOD: For time

100 Double unders
800m walk with plate over head (20/15)
200m walk with 2 plates in pinch grip (15/10)
400 m walk with plate overhead
200m walk with 2 plates in pinch grip
100 double unders

session 516

strength/skill:
20 min to find bench press 1rm

WOD: AMRAP 20 min

O/H lunge x 10 (5 each leg 50/35)
HSPU x 7
burpee muscle up x 4

session 517

strength/skill:
20 min to find deadlift 1RM

WOD: FRAN
21/15/9
thruster (40/30)
pull up

session 518

strength/skill:
15 min to find power clean 1RM

WOD: Bear complex

5 rounds for load
7 x power clean/front squat/push press/back squat/push press

bar must not rest on ground, it may rest in rack position or on back or in hang.
rest as need between rounds

session 519

12 days of xmas

Following the theme of the song
1
2,1
3,2,1
4,3,2,1 etc….

1 x cluster (60/40)
2 x muscle ups
3 x thrusters
4 x bar facing burpees

5 x hang power cleans
6 x wallballs
7 x toes to bar
8 x kb snatch (4 each arm 20/16)
9 x goblet squats (20/16)
10 x kb swings
11x push ups
12 x front rack lunges

 session 520
strength/skill:

EMOM: 7 min
power clean/ 2 x front squat

EMOM: 7 min
hang squat clean/ front squat x 1

EMOM: 7 min
full clean

rest 2 min between each emom.

WOD: 10 min ascending ladder
burpee pull up
thruster (30/40)

session 521

strength/skill:
bench press 3 x 8

WOD: 3 rounds

21x push up
15 x kb snatch each arm (20/16)
9 x burpee

session   522

strength/skill:

back squat 3 x 8
paused back squat 3 x 2 (5 sec pause)

WOD: 3 rounds
 AMRAP - 3 min
400m run
wall balls in remainder

rest 2 min

session 523

strength/skill:
strict press 3 x 8
push press 3 x 5

WOD: 2 rounds for time
30 x burpee box jump
30 x pull up
30 x ring dip
30 x sumo high pull (40/30)

session 524
mash

session 525

strength/skill:
deadlift 5 x 5

WOD: AMRAP 8 min

push up x 12
sit up x 15

session 526

strength/skill:
rope climbs

WOD: ELIZABETH

21/15/9
clean (60/40)
ring dips

session 527

strength/skill:
front squat 6 x 4

WOD:
12/9/6/3

HSPU
Muscle up
TTB

session 528

strength/skill:
hang power snatch 5 x 3

WOD: AMRAP 15 min
double under x 30
air squat x 40
squat snatch x 1 (60/40)

session 529

strength/skill:
strict pull up 5 x 12-15

WOD: 4 Rounds

sumo high pulls x 10 (60/40)
400m run

session 530
mash

session 531

strengthg/skill:
bench press 5 x 5

WOD:
1 min on, 1 min off
4 rounds

first minute - burpee to target
second minute - jumping lunges with wall ball

session 532

strength/skill:
power clean - 3/3/2/2/1/1

 3 x max effort hang power clean @ 80% of highest set from above

WOD: open WOD 13.4

AMRAP - 7 min
ascending ladder 3/6/9/12 etc…

clean and jerk (60/40)
TTB

session 533

strength/skill:
back squat 5 x 5

WOD: Open WOD 12.1

AMRAP 7 min
burpees

session 534

strength/skill:
ring dips 5 x max effort

WOD: Open WOD 12.4
AMRAP 12 min
150 x wallballs
90 x double unders
30 x muscle ups

session 535

strength/skill:
deadlift 5 x 5

WOD: open WOD 14.1

AMRAP 10 min

30 x double unders
15 x snatch (30/20)

session 536

mash

session 537

strength/skill:
O/H squat - 3 x 3

WOD: for time
30 x snatch (40/30)
30 x clean and jerk
30 x thruster
30 x bar facing burpee

session 538

strength/skill:
weighted pull up 5 x 3

WOD: Open WOD   15.4

AMRAP 8 min
HSPU
Cleans (85/55)

rep scheme-

h	c
3	3
6	3
9	3
12	6
15	6
18	6
21	9
24	9
27	9

session   539

strength/skill:
split jerk 5 x 2

WOD:
21/15/9/6/3
front squat (60/40)
push ups (double reps)

session 540
mash

session 541

strength/skill:
bench press 4 x 8
superset with
bent over rows

WOD: AMRAP 16 min
5 x pull up
10 x dips
15 x wallball
20 x lunges

session 542

strength/skill:
EMOM 10 min
power clean/hang power clean/ full clean

3 min rest

EMOM 10 min
cluster from hang x 2

WOD: for time
400m run
10 x muscle up
20 x cluster (60/40)
10 x muscle up
400 m run

session 543

Hero WOD murph

1.6 km run
100 pull ups
200 push ups
300 squats
1.6 km run

(you may partition up the push/pull ups and squats)

session 544

strength/skill:

push jerk - work up to a heavy single

emom 6 min - 2 x push jerk @ 80-85%

WOD: AMRAP 8 min
9 x deadlift (60/40)
9 x burpee box jump

rest 2 min

AMRAP 5 min
5 x wall ball
5 x kb push press (each arm 20/16)

session 545

strength/skill:
accumulate 3 min in
L-sit and hand stand (may use wall)

WOD: 5 rounds
20 x deadstart kb snatch (20/16)
15 x shoulder to overhead (60/40)
10 x hang power clean

session 546
mash

session 547

strength/skill:
deadlift 4 x 8

WOD: ascending EMOM
3,6,9,12…. etc until failure
med ball clean

rest
then

tabata hollow rock

session 548

strength/skill:
work up to a heavy power snatch single

then
EMOM 5 min 2 x power snatch @ 80-85%

WOD 3 rounds for time

21 x push up
15 x TTB
9 x power snatch (50/35)

session 549

strength/skill:
front squat 4 x 4
front squat (1 and 1/4) 3 x 5

WOD: For time

6/9/12/15/12/9/6

thruster (40/30)
box jump

session   550

strength/skill:
Hang power clean - 3/3/2/2/2

WOD - for time
5/10/15
power clean (70/50)
push jerk
wallball (reps x3)

session 551

strength/skill:
EMOM 10 min
7 x pull up, 7 x dips

WOD: For time

walking lunge x 100 (60/40)
EMOM - 5 x burpees

session 552
mash

session 553

strength/skill:
close grip bench press- 10/10/8/8/6

WOD: AMRAP- 20 min
as partners
run 400m
deadlift x 80 (60/40)
HR push up x 60
Knees to elbows x 40
burpee x 20

session 554

strength/skill:
3 sets of max effortt pull ups

WOD: 5 Rounds for time
KB swings x 30 (20/16)
muscle up x 7
run 200m

session 555

strength/skill:
deadlift work up to a 3rm

every 90 secs for 6 rounds - 2 reps at 3rm weight

WOD: 3 rounds
AMRAP 5 min
o/h squat x 9 (40/30)
TTB x 7
hang power snatch x 5
rest 2 min

session 556

strength/skill:
back squat- 8 x 3

WOD: AMRAP 3 min
HR push up x 8
KB sumo high pull x 8 (20/16)

session 557

strength/skill:
bent over row - 10 x 10 (3 sec negative) 45 sec rest between sets

WOD: 5 rounds for time

50 x double under
10 x burpee pull up

session 558
mash

session 559

strength/skill:
turkish get up 5 x 5 each side

WOD: 3 rounds

0.00-2.00
400 m run
max double unders

2:00- 3:00
kb push jerk (20/16)

3:00- 4:00
push ups

4:00-5:00
med ball cleans
rest 3 min between rounds

session 560

strength/skill:
EMOM 21 min
1- pull up x 10
2- hang power clean x 5
3- full clean and jerk x 2

WOD: AMRAP - 5 min
double under x 30
air squat x 15

session 561
strength/skill:
HSPU - 3 x 10
or
accumulate 3min in handstand

WOD: filthy 50
50 of each movement

box jumps
jumping pull ups
kb swing (16/12)
walking lunge
knees to elbow
push press (20/15)
back extension
wallballs

burpees
double unders

session 562

strength/skill:
legless or L-sit rope climbs - 6 ascents

WOD: For time

30 x sit ups
15 x squat clean (70/50)
24 x sit ups
12 x squat clean
18 x sit ups
9 x squat clean
12 x sit ups
6 x squat clean
6 x sit ups
3 x squat clean

session 563

strength/skill:
4 x complex of - 4 strict press/ 3 push press/ 2 push jerk/ split jerk

WOD: For time

800m run
power snatch x 10 (50/35)
400m run
power snatch x 10
200m run
thruster x 10
100m run
thruster x 10

session 564
monster mash

For time as a 2 person team:
400 Double - unders

200 Ring dips
100 Squat cleans 100/70
50 Rope climbs, 15 ft
*Divide the reps between the partners as desired. All double-unders must be completed before beginning dips. All dips before cleans. All cleans before rope climbs.

session 565

strength/skill:
bench press 5x5

WOD- AMRAP 7 min

kb push press x 5 each arm (20/12)
kb goblet squat x 10 (alternating)
kb swing x 15

session 566

open wod 16.1

session 567

strength/skill:
push press 5 x 3

WOD :AMRAP 8 min
9 x burpee box over
9 x push press (60/40)
9 x ring dips

session 568

strength/skill:
snatch - 4 x 1
snatch pull - 3 x 3

WOD: 3 rounds for time
TTB x 20
squat snatch x 5 (50/35)
O/H squat x 5

session 569

strength/skill:
Muscle ups

WOD: 5 rounds of max front squats in 30 secs @ 60% of 1rm
rest 2:30 between rounds

3 rounds of max hang power clean in 30 secs @ 60 % of 1rm
rest 1:30 between rounds

3 rounds of max double unders in 30 secs, 30 secs rest

session 570

mash

session 571

strength/skill:
accumulate 3 min in L-sit and 3 min in support position (top of dip with
externally rotated arms)

WOD:
12 rounds of each for time

1 x deadlift (120/80)
6 x bar hops

1 x HSPU
6 x bar hops

1 x L-sit pull up
2 x bar hop burpees

1 x thruster (50/35)
2 x bar hop burpees

session 572
open wod 16.2

session 573

strength/skill:
bench press 4 x 10

WOD: for time
40/30/20
box jumps
wallballs
jumping lunges

session 574
strength/skill:
power clean 5 x 2

WOD: AMRAP 12 min

C2B x 8
man makers x 10 (15/7.5)

session 575

strength/skill:
O/H squat 4 x 10

WOD: 5 rounds each for time

thrusters x 15 (40/30)
DB snatch x 12 (20/15)
burpee x 10

rest 3 min

session   576

mash and 16.2

session 577

16.2

session 578

strength/skill:
front squat- 2/2/2/1/1/1

WOD: for time
30 burpee muscle ups
or
50 burpee pull ups

session 579

strength/skill: front lever

WOD: 5 rounds for time

10 x push press (50/35)
10 x sumo high pull
10 x hang power clean

session 580
strength/skill:
Back squat - 20/15/10

WOD: for time
100m walk with plates in pinch grip (15/10)

20 x db alternating dumbbell snatch (20/15)

200m walk with plates
30 x dumbbell snatch

400m walk with plates
40 x dumbbell snatch

session 581
mash

session 582

strength/skill:
O/H lungres 5 x 10m

WOD: 20 min chelsea

EMOM 20 min
5 x pull up
10 x push up
15 x squat

session 583
open wid 16.4

session 584
strength/skill:
clean and jerk 4 x 3

WOD: AMRAP 12 min

TTB x 12
box jump x 15
DB squat x 12 (20/15)

session 584

strength/skill:
push press - 5/3/3/2/2

WOD:
buy in- 400m run
buy out - 20 burpees

3 rounds for time
10 x ring dip
15 x HR push up
45 x double unders

session 585

strength/skill:

strength:
front squat 5 x 5

WOD: 4 x 500m row

session 586
16.5

session 587

strength/skill:
hang power snatch 5 x 2

WOD: Dianne

21/15/9

Deadlift (100/70)
hspu

session 588
strength/skill:

bench press - 4 x 7

WOD: AMRAP 15 min

push up x 50
KB swing x 50 (20/16)
ring dip x 50
box jump x 50

session   589

strength/skill:
EMOM - 12 min
2 x (power clean/ push jerk)
rest 2 min
EMOM - 6 min
squat clean / push jerk

WOD: AMRAP 10 min

TTB x 8
Hang power clean x 6 (70/45)

session 590
mash

session 591

strength/skill:
front rack lunge
20m/15m/10m/6m/6m/6m

WOD: AMRAP 6 min
kb sumo high pull x 12 (20/16)
double under x 20

rest 3 min

AMRAP 6 min
db push press x 8 (20/15)
KTE x 8

session 592

strength/skill:
back squat 10/8/6/3/3/3

WOD:
AMRAP 8 min
12 x hspu
15 x pull up

session 593

strength/skill:
strict press 5 x 5
push press 5 x 1 (3 sec pause in dip)

WOD: AMRAP 8 min

30 wallballs
20 burpees

session 594

strength/skill:
sumo highpull 4 x 3

WOD: 3 rounds each for time

120 x double under
10 x clean and jerk (70/45)
8 x bar muscle up

rest 2 min between rounds

session 595
strength/skill:

deadlift 3 x 10

WOD: for time

AMRAP 15 min

air squat x 100
burpee x 20
DB thruster x 50 (20/15)
burpee x 20

session 596
mash

session 597
strength/skill:
bench press 3 x 10
DB bench press 3 x 12

WOD: 2 rounds for reps

60 sec at each station

box jump
wallball
double unders
front rack lunges with ball

rest 1 min

1 round for reps

session 598

strength/skill:
O/H squat - 5 x 3

WOD: for time

hang power snatch x 25 (40/25)

burpee x 20
thruster x 25
burpee x 20
hang power snatch x 25

session 599

strength/skill:
front squat complex
1- 1 @ (50x0)
2- 1 @ 3 sec pause at parallel on concentric,
3- 2 @(10x0)

complete 5 sets increasing load each set

WOD:
4 Rounds
14 x alternating DB snatch (20/15)
14 x pull up
28 x double under

session 600

600th WOD!

3 Rounds for time

5 x deadlift (120/80)
10 x burpee over bar
20 x box jump
30 x wall ball
40 x sit up
30 x jumping lunges
20 x air squat
10 x kb sumo high pull (20/16)
5 x dips

session 601

strength/skill:

push press 5/5/3/3/3/2/2

WOD: AMRAP 7 min
DB squat x 8 (20/15)
DB over head lunge x 10

session 602
mash

session 603

strength/skill:
turkish get ups
5 x 5 each arm

WOD: 10-1
burpee pull up
wallball

*turkish get up each arm every 2 min (12/8)

session 604

strength/skill:
10 min to find a 2RM "touch and go" clean
then
EMOM 4 min
2 touch and go cleans at 85% of above

WOD: 21/15/9/6/3
hang squat clean (60/40)
pull up

session 605

strength/skill:
dips 5 x 5 weighted

WOD:
DU x 100
HSPU x 2
DU's x 80
HSPU x 4
DU's x 60
HSPU x 6
DU's x 40
HSPU x 8
DU's x 20
HSPU x 10

session 606

strength/skill:
deadlift 5 x 3

WOD:
tabata
air squat
push press (40/30)

1 min rest

tabata
push up
hang power clean (40/30)

session 607
strength/skill:
front lunges 5 x 10m

WOD: for time
50 x thrusters (40/30)
40 x TTB
30 x O/H squat
20 x box jumps
10 x shoulder to O/H
5 x rounds of cindy

session 608
mash

session 609
strength/skill:
strict press 3 x 5
db push press 3 x 10 (one arm at a time)

WOD: 30/20/10
bench press (60/40)
broad jumps

session 610
strength/skill:
front squat - 7 x 2

WOD: AMRAP 7 min
kb swing x 12 (20/12)
100m sprint

session 611

strength/skill:
pull up 5 x 5 weighted

WOD: for time
cluster x 15 (60/40)
cindy x 5
cluster x 10
cindy x 4
cluster x 5
cindy x 3

session 612

strength/skill:
20 min to find 1RM bench press
or
5 x 5

WOD:
AMRAP 6 min
15 burpees
10 push press (30/20)

session 613
mash

session 614

strength/skill:
ring row 5 x 10 (horizontal as possible)

WOD:
in 4 min complete-
20 x kb swing (20/12)
400m run
amrap double unders in remaining time.

rest 3 min
repeat for 4 rounds

session 615

strength/skill:
find heaviest complex of - power clean/hang squat clean
then
EMOM 7 min
above complex at 85%

WOD: 3 rounds for time

15 x power clean (60/40)
400m farmers walk (20/15 db's)

session 616

strength/skill:
push jerk 6/4/2/6/4/2

WOD: 15 min clock
3 - box jumps
3 - wallballs
10 - HR push ups

6 - box jumps
6 - wallballs
10 - HR push ups

9 - box jumps
9 - wallballs
10 - HR push ups

increase box jump/wallball reps by 3 each round

session   617

WOD: masters league workout #2

12 min clock

50 cal row

21/15/9
ground to overhead (42/30)
TTB/Knee raise

amrap of cal row in remaining time

session 618

strength/skill:
thruster - 3/3/2/2/1/1 (rack is allowed)

WOD: 3 rounds each for time
24 x thrusters (40/30)
24 x pull ups

24 x DB power snatch (20/15)

rest 3 min

session 619
mash

session 620

strength/skill:
Ring dips - 3 x max effort

WOD: amrap 7 min

Double under x 50
back squat x 10 (60/40)

rest 2 min

amrap 5 min
100m sprint
front squat x 8 (50/35)

rest 1 min

amrap 3 min
burpee x 6
O/H squat x 6 (40/30)

session 621

strength:
front squat 5 x 8

WOD:
104 x wallball
52 x pull up

session 623

strength/skill:
every 90 sec for 10 rounds
1 x squat clean
1 x thruster
1 x split jerk

WOD: 4 rounds for time

28 x jumping lunges
15 x power clean (50/35)

sesssion 624

masters leauge 16.3

Running clock
3 rounds of
12 x deadlift (80/60)
16 x KB swing
20 x HR pushup

into

1km run
2 rounds of
15 x snatch (40/30)
20 x wallballs

session 625

strength/skill:
bench press 5 x 8
super set
DB row

WOD: in pairs complete for time

200 x sit up
150 x box jump
100 x bench press (60/35)
50 x Toes to rings

session   626

mash

session 627

strength/skill:
DB over head squat 5 x 5

WOD:
4 x 5 min rounds

18 x DB squats (20/15)
9x DB push jerk

14 x DB squat
7 x DB push jerk

10 x DB squat
5 x DB push jerk

6 x DB squat
3 x DB push jerk

amrap burpees in remaining time
rest 2 min

session 628

strength/skill:
squat snatch - find heavy single

WOD: 2 rounds for time

40 x push ups

30 x O/H squat (40/30)
20 x hang power clean
10 x burpee

session 629

strength/skill:
EMOM 18 min
min 1- 10-15 pull ups
min 2 - 10-15 dips
min 3 - 5 x push jerk (no rack allowed)

WOD: AMRAP 8 min
6 x sumo high pull (60/40)
30 x double under

session 630

masters wod 16.4

12 min AMRAP

21/15/9

front squat (50/35)
bar facing burpee
Double under 60/80/100

amrap of chest to bar pull ups in remainder time

strait into 3 min squat clean ladder

must complete 5 reps at designated weight before increasing.
50/30
60/40
70/50
80/60
90/70
100/80

session 631

strength/skil:
EMOM - 14 min
min 1- 2 x power clean @ 70-80% , 15 x double under
min 2 - 4 x burpee pull up

WOD: 15 rounds for time
2 x deadlift (150/ 100)
5 x box jump

session 632
mash

session 633

WOD: EMOM
5 x front squat

guys start at 30 kg
girls start at 20 kg

guys increase weight buy 10kg every 5th round
girls increase weight by 5kg every 5th round

session 634

strength/skill:
hang power snatch 3 x 3
snatch deadlift 3 x 3 (5 sec eccentric)

WOD: AMRAP 7 min
TTB x 12
front rack db lunges x 12 (6 each leg @ 20/15)

session 635
strength/skill:
EMOM 10 min - strict c2b x 5-8

WOD: 5 x 5 min round

round 1 - 200m run then 50 wall balls
round 2 - (starts at 5 min mark) 200 m run then 40 deadlifts (50/35)
round 3- (starts at 10min) 200m run then 30 hang power clean
round 4- (starts at 15min) 200m run then 20 push jerks
round 5 - (starts at 20min) 200m run then 10 thrusters

session 636

strength/skill:
back squat - 5 x 5

WOD: 2 rounds for time
20 x kb swing (20/16)
10 x front squat (70/45)
15 x burpee

strait into

50 x DB power snatch (20/15)*
*5 burpees every 10 snatches

session 637
strength/skill:
work up to heaviest complex of
cluster/push press/split jerk

then EMOM for 8 min of above complex @ 80-85%

WOD: 3 rounds for time

24 x push press (40/30)
12 x dips
400m run

session 638
mash

session 639
strength/skill:

O/H squat - 5 x 2 (3 sec pause at bottom)

WOD: for time

5/4/3/2/1
power clean (100/65)
100/80/60/40/20
double unders

session 640
amrap 6 min
10 x dips
15 x kb swing
20 x air squat

at 10 min
6 min amrap
1000m row
max burpees

at 20min
6 min amrap
3 x bar muscle up
25 x jumping squat

at 30min
6 min amrap
20 x wall ball
10 x TTB

at 40min

6 min amrap
12 x plate thruster (20/15)
10 x push up

session 641

strength/skill:
weighted dips 5 x 5
super set
max effort strict pull ups

WOD: 4 x 3 min amrap
15 hspu
max effort cluster in remaining

1st round (40/30)
2nd round (50/35)
3rd round (60/40)
4th round (70/45)

1 min rest between rounds

session   642

strength/skill:
bench press 5 x 5

WOD: 4 rounds for time

400m run
6 x deadlift (125/80)

session 643
mash

session 643

strength/skill:
EMOM- 21 min

1- row for cal (15/12)
2- 6 x front squat (60/40)
3- 4 x burpee box step over with DB's (15/7.5)

WOD: 3 rounds for time

27 x double under
21 x KB sumo high pull (20/16)
15 x DB thruster (20/15)

session 642

strength/skill:
push press - 1/6/1/6/1/6
aim is 90%,75%,92%,77.5%,95%,80%

WOD: for time
400m farmers walk
30 x overhead squat (60/40)
20 x burpee muscle up
10 x power snatch

session 643
strength/skill:
3 sets of complex - hang squat clean/power clean/hang power clean

WOD: amrap 20 min
5 x chest to bar pull ups
10 x ring dips
15 x squat clean (40/30)

session 644

strength/skill:
push ups on rings - 4 x max effort
ring rows - 4 max effort

WOD: 21/15/9
box jump
TTB

rest 3 min

then "grace"
30 x clean and jerks (60/40)

session 645

strength/skill:
back squat - 6 x 4

WOD: amrap 6 min
12 x DB power snatch
12 x wallball

session 646
mash

session 647

strength/skill:
bench press - 3 x 12

WOD: for time
200 x walking lunges with KB in rack (16/12)
*must perform 10 x swing and 3 burpees every time KB leaves rack

session 648

strength/skill:
muscle up

WOD: DT
5 rounds for time
12 x deadlift (70/50)
9 x hang power clean
6 x push jerk

rest 5 min

Tabata Assault bike

session 649
strength/skill:
1 RM strict press

3 x 5 strict press @ 75- 80% of above

WOD: amrap 1 min
thrusters (40/30)
30 sec rest

amrap 1 min
front squat
rest 30 sec

amrap 1 min
push press

2 min rest

repeat for 3 rounds

session 650
mash

session 651

strength/skill:
back squat 3 x 12
front squat 1 1/2s - 3 x 5

WOD: EMOM 20 min
1- DB snatch x 12
2- burpee x 12

session 652

strength/skill:
snatch balance - 5 x 3

WOD: 21/15/9/15/21

DB push jerk (20/15)
pull up

session   653

strength/skill:

EMOM: 7 min
power clean/ 2 x front squat

EMOM: 7 min
hang squat clean/ front squat

EMOM: 7 min
full clean

rest 2 min between each emom.

WOD: AMRAP 9 min

Kb swing x 10
burpee x 5
Kb swing x 20
burpee x 10
Kb swing x 30
burpee x 15
Kb swing x 40
burpee x 20
Kb swing x 50
burpee x 25
Continue pattern untill 9 min is up

session 654

strength/skill:

EMOM: 7 min
power clean/ 2 x front squat

EMOM: 7 min

hang squat clean/ front squat

EMOM: 7 min
full clean

rest 2 min between each emom.

WOD: AMRAP 9 min

Kb swing x 10
burpee x 5
Kb swing x 20
burpee x 10
Kb swing x 30
burpee x 15
Kb swing x 40
burpee x 20
Kb swing x 50
burpee x 25
Continue pattern untill 9 min is up
21/6/16

session 655

strength/skill:
weighted pull ups 5 x 5

WOD: AMRAP 18 min
muscle up x 6
deadlift x 12 (100/70)
box jump x 18
TTB x 24

session 656
mash

session 657
strength/skill:
thruster - 5 x 3

WOD: 5 x 1 min max effort assault bike for cals

session 658

strength/skill:
back squat 3 x 3
paused back squat 3 x 3 (pause at parallel)

WOD: AMRAP 12 min
ascending reps (1 a side, 2 a side, 3 a side etc)
db snatch (20/15)
jumping lung with med ball

session 659
strength/skill:
bench press - 10/8/6
super set with max effort ring dips

WOD: for time
15/12/9/6/3

thruster (50/35)
25 double unders between rounds

session 670

strength/skill:
hang power clean - 5/4/3/2/1

WOD: amrap - 2 min
sumo high pull x 12 (40/30)
box jump x 24
pull up x 12
hang power clean x 24

rest 2 min
repeat as 3 min amrap

rest 2 min
repeat for time

session 671

strength/skill:
front squat - emom
4 min - 4 @ 70%
4 min - 3 @ 80%
3 min - 1-2 @ 90%

WOD: 25 rounds for time
1 x strict muscle up
2 x squat clean (80/55)
3 x hspu

session 672
mash

session 678

strength/skill:
deadlift work up to a heavy double
then
every 90 secs for 5 rounds
3 @ 80% of above

WOD: AMRAP 10 min
burpee x 6
Knees to elbows x 8
air squat x 10

session 679
strength/skill:
snatch balance - 5 x 3
or OH squat 5 x 3

WOD: AMRAP 8 min
8 x wallball
8 x OH DB lunges right arm (20/15)
8 x OH DB lunges left arm

session 680

strength/skill:
2 RM push press

WOD: "bergeron beep test"
EMOM as long as possible

7 x thruster (30/25)
7 x burpee
7 x pull up

30 min cap

session 681

strength/skill:
deadlift - 2/5/2/5/2/5

WOD:
500m row
strait into
2 min max cals on bike

session 682

strength/skill:
E2MOM - 14 min
power clean/ clean/ 2 x front squat

WOD - for time
30/20/10
KB snatch (24/16)
deficit push up (6"/3")
pull up

session 683
mash

session 694

strength/skill:
DB snatch- work to heavy single
then
emom 12 min
1- db snatch x 3 each arm
2- push up x 10-15

WOD: AMRAP - 12 min
1 x db snatch each arm (20/15)
20 x air squat
20 x sit up

2 x db snatch each arm
20 x air squat
20 x sit up

3 x db snatch each arm
20 x air squat
20 x sit up

continue adding a rep to snatches until time is up

session 685

strength/skill:
1RM thruster

WOD: fran
21/15/9
thruster (42.5/30)
pull up

sessoin 686

strength/skill:
strict pull up - 4 sets (aim is 12-15)
super set
bent over row x 10-15 @ 50% of clean

WOD: for time
30 x hspu
60 x double under
30 x OH squat (40/30)
60 x double under
30 x man maker (20/15)

session 687

strength/skill:
dips - 4 sets max effort
super set
db bench press (12-15 reps)

WOD: "karen"
150 wallballs
rest 3 min
50 x db hang squat clean (20/15)

session 688

strength/skill:
push jerk - 5 x 3

WOD- 3 rounds for time
10 x clean and jerk (50/35)
20 x TTB

session 1689
mash

session 690

strength/skill:
bench press 5 x 5

WOD: "angie"
100 of each

pull up
push up
sit ups
squats

session 691

strength/skill:
hang squat snatch - work up to a heavy double

WOD: AMRAP 4 min
3 x power clean (60/40)

6 x hspu
9 x air squat
rest 1 min

repeat for 4 rounds

session 692

strength/skill:
front squat 5 x 2

WOD: for time
kb swing x 30 (28/20)
assault bike for cals (40/30)
jumping lunge x 20

session 693

strength/skill: muscle up

WOD: 5 rounds for time

double under x 50
push press x 10 (40/30)
muscle up x 5

session 694
strength/skill:
deadlift 3 x 2 @ 83-87%
then
4 rounds
3 speed reps every 90 secs @ 70%

WOD: 15/12/9
burpee box jump
burpee pull up

session 695
mash

session 696

strength/skill:
strict press 3 x 8

WOD:

tabata - wallball
rest 3 min
tabata - row
rest 3 min
tabata - burpee
rest 3 min
tabata - hollow rock

session 697

strength/skill:
for load-
new round every 3 min for 5 rounds, 1 round of "DT"
start light and aim for a max effort in the last round.

WOD: for time
50 bar over burpees
50 O/H lunge steps (50/35)

session 698

strength/skill:
split jerk 5 x 1

WOD: DB "fran"
21/15/9
db thrusters
pull ups

session 699

strength/skill:
EMOM- 10 min
power snatch / full snatch

WOD: amrap 3 min
burpee box overs x 4
power snatch x 4 (40/30)

rest 2 min

amrap 3 min
wallballs x 6
TTB x 6

rest 2 min

amrap 6 min
burpee box over x 4
power snatch x 4
wallball x 6
TTB x 6

session 700
heavy day - back squat 1/2/3/1/2/3/1/2/3

session 701
mash

session 702
strength/skill:
single arm DB squat clean - 5 x 3 Each arm

WOD: 25 min KB carry for distance (24/20)
Kb may be held how ever but must not touch ground, aim is to keep in rack position.
*5 swings every minute

session 703

strength/skill:
EMOM- 14 min
1- 3 x power cleans (90/60)
2- 12 x C2B

WOD: in 2 teams row as far as possible in 20 min
swapping every 300m

session 704

strength/skill:

O/H squat - find heavy single
then 3 x 2 @ 88-90%

WOD: for time
100 x O/H squat (20/15)
100 x thrusters
*5 burpees every 2 min
*Rx+ 5 burpees every min

session 705
strength/skill:
weighted dips 5 x 5 (drop weight after 5th rep and continue till failure)

WOD: 3 rounds for time
20 x wallball
20 x box jump
20 x sumo high pull (40/30)

session 706

strength/skill:
find heavy complex of:
power clean/ push press x3/ push jerk x2

WOD: ascending ladder 12 min
deadlift x 1 (140/100)
double unders x 10

deadlift increase 1 rep each round
double under increase x 10

session 707
mash

session 708

strength/skill:
bench press 5 x 5

WOD: 21/15/9
KB swing (28/20)
push press (40/30)

session 709
strength/skill:
5 sets of - squat clean/ 4 x lunge/ squat clean/ 4 x lunge

WOD: 10-1
wallball
DB snatch (20/15)

session 723

strength/skill:
snatch balance 5 x 2

WOD: for time
800m run
100 x push up
10 x squat snatch (60/40)

session 724

strength/skill:
deadlift 5 x 5

if time allows

WOD: 1 min max effort cals on bike

session 726

strength/skill:
strict press- 4 x 7

WOD: Annie
50/40/30/20/10
sit ups
double unders

session 727

strength/skill:
find heaviest- 2 x front squat / split jerk

WOD: 3 rounds for time
20 x pistol squat
15 x hspu
10 x box jump overs
5 x muscle up

session 728

strength/skill:
pendlay rows 5 x 5

WOD: amrap 12 min
ascending reps 2/4/6/8…etc
TTB
power cleans (60/40)

session 729
strength/skill:
pistol squats

WOD:
4 x 500m row

session 731
mash

session 732
strength/skill:
bench press 3 x 10

WOD: 3 rounds for time

400 m run
25 kb swings (24/16)
15 burpees

session 733
strength/skill:
back squat 5 x 2 (4,3,x,0)

WOD: AMRAP 8 min
muscle snatch x 8 (40/25)
bar over burpee

session 734

strength/skill:
clean and jerk - 3/3/2/2/1/1

WOD: 15/9/6
DB clusters (20/15)
C2B pull ups

session 735

strength/skill:
muscle up

WOD: 10-1
hang power snatch (50/35)
O/H squat
muscle up

session 736

strength/skill:
single arm DB push press - 5 x 5 each arm

WOD: amrap 4 min
wallball x 18
TTB x 9

rest 2 min

AMRAP 4 min
burpee pull up

rest 2 min

AMRAP 8 min
wallball x 50
TTB x 35

burpee pull up in remaining time

session 737
mash

session 738

strength/skill:
hang power clean - 5 x 2

WOD: AMRAP - 12
min
30 x burpee
30 x air squat
30 x jumping lunge

session 739
strength/skill:
push press 3 x 3

WOD: for time
100 x double under
50 x push up
30 x DB snatch alternating (20/15)
10 x bar muscle up
30 x DB snatch
50 x push up
100 x double under

session 740
strength/skill:
EMOM - 5 min
3 x squat clean

rest 3 min

EMOM - 5 min
2 x squat clean

rest 3 min

EMOM - 5 min
1 x squat clean

WOD: Dianne
21/15/9
deadlift (102/70)
hspu

session 741
strength/skill
bench press- 5 x 3

WOD: 3 rounds for time
12 x kb clean and jerk right arm (24/16)
12 x clean and jerk left arm
10 x O/H lunge right arm
10 x O/H lunge left arm

session 742

strength/skill:
pull ups

WOD: 5 RFT
10 x push press (50/35)
200 m run

session 743

strength/skill:
O/H squat - 5 x 2 (3,3,x,0)

WOD: AMRAP 9 min

100 double under buy in
then
amrap in remaining
HR push up x 10
box jump x 12
wallball x 14

session 744

strength/skill:
5 x complex
3 x strict press/ 2 x push press/ push jerk

WOD: helen
3 rounds
400m run
21 x kb swing (24/16)
12 x pull up

session 745

strength/kill:
deadlift - 3/3/2/2/1/1

WOD: in teams 10min max cals on bike
person that is riding must keep bike over (80/65rpm) once rpm is lost switch
riders

session 746

strength/skill:
push ups on rings 5 x 10-15

WOD: 7 rounds for time

7 x thruster (50/35)
7 x hspu
7 x TTB
7 x hang power clean

session 747
mash

session 748

strength/skill:
front squat - 3 x 5

WOD:
tabata- plate thruster (20/15)
rest 2 min
tabata - Knees to elbow

rest 1 min

3 rounds for time

21 jumping lunges with med ball (20/14)
12 burpees

session 750

strength/skill:
strict press - 10/8/6/4/2

WOD: amrap 5 min
ring dips x 30
kb snatches in remainder (24/16)

rest 2 min

AMRAP 5 min
pull up x 30
kb clean and jerk in remainder

rest 2 min

AMRAP 5 min
muscle up x 10
KB swing in remainder

session 751

strength/skill:
20 min to find 1rm pull up
or
5 sets of max effort

WOD: 10-1
deadlift (120/80)
burpee box over

session 752
front squat 4 reps, 2 @ (4,4,x,2) 2 @ (1,0,x,1)
complete 4 sets

WOD: for time
20 x thrusters (45/32.5)

20 x sumo high pull
20 x push jerk
20 x OH squat
20 x front squat

5 burpees at the start of each minute

session 753

strength/skill:
squat clean 3/3/2/2/1/1
3 sec pause at knee and in squat

WOD: amrap 9 min
ascending ladder - 3,6,9,12 etc....
db thruster (20/15)
burpee

session 754

strength/skill:
push press - 3 x 3
DB strict press 3 x 10 each arm

WOD: 10 rounds for time
3 x sumo high pull (60/40)
9 x HR push up
27 x double under

session 755

strength/skill:
hang squat snatch - work to heavy single

WOD: for time

50 x KB swings (28/20)
40 x O/H squat (40/30)
30 x Hang power clean
20 x pull up
10 x TTB
20 x pull up
30 x hang power clean
40 x O/H squat

50 x KB swing

session 756

strength/skill:
front rack lunge 5 x 12m

WOD: 12 min amrap

left arm overhead DB lunge x 15
right arm OH lunge x 15
ring dip x 10

session 759

strength/skill:
power clean 2 reps every 90 seconds for 7 rounds

WOD:
21/15/9
front squat (70/50)
box jump

session 760

strength/skill:
sumo high pull 5 x 3

WOD: AMRAP 3 min
kb swing x 12 (24/12)
kb snatch x 6 each arm
kb clean and jerk x 6 each arm
rest 90 sec

repeat x 3

rest 1 min

100 push ups for time

session 761

strength/skill:
thruster - 3rm

then 3 x 2 @ 90% of 3rm

WOD:
5 rounds
24 x double under
12 x db hang squat clean (20/15)
6 x db shoulder to overhead

session 762

strength/skill:
work up to heavy complex of -
snatch push press x 3/ overhead squat x 3

or
5 x 3 O/H squat

WOD: AMRAP 17 min

hang power snatch x 3 (60/40)
muscle up x 5
hspu x 7

session 763
mash

session 764

strength/skill:
back squat - 20/15/10/5
follow every set imeadiately with 3 box jumps

WOD: emom- 21 min
min 1- db snatch x 12
min 2 - pull up x 12
min 3 - burpee x 12

session 766
strength/skill:
back squat- 15 min to find a 2RM
then
3 x 2 @ 90-95% of above

WOD: AMRAP 8 min
back squat @ 80% of 1RM

1 min rest

AMRAP 90 seconds
burpees

30 sec rest

AMRAP 1 min
plate snatch (20/15)

session 767
19/10/16

strength/skill:
EMOM 4 min - hang power clean x 2 @75%+
2 min rest
EMOM 4 min - hang power clean x 1 @ 85%+

WOD: for time

30 wallballs
30 TTB
30 clean and jerk (60/40)
30 TTB
30 wallballs

session 768

WOD:

10 alternating DB snatch (20/15)
90 sec row sprint
10 DB snatch

perform 10 rounds resting as need between efforts.
score is time of round and meters rowed.

session 769
mash

session 770

WOD: double under chelsea

emom 30 min
5 x pull up
10 x push up
15 x air squat
double unders in remaining time

score is round with most double unders

session 772

strength/ skill:
AHAP
4 sets of - push press + split jerk

WOD: 30/20/10
push press (50/35)
bar over burpee

session 773

strength/skill:
deadlift 5 x 5 @78%

WOD: ascending ladder 8 min
2/4/6/8..etc
renegade rows
pull ups

session 774

strength/skill:
ring dip 3 x max effort

WOD: 10 rounds for time
20 - 11 of wallballs
10 - 1 of TTB
25 double unders after each round

session 775
mash

session 776

strength/skill:
db snatch 5 x 3 each arm

WOD: emom - 21 min
1 - kb swing x 20 (24/16)
2 - 100m sprint
3 - 10 x burpee broad jump

session 777

strength/skill:
back squat 5 x 5

wod amrap 9 min
kte x 12
burpee x 9
oh squat x 12

session 778

strength/skill:
strict pull pull up 3 x max effort

WOD: 5 rounds for time

400m run
25 x wallballs
15 x push ups

session 779
mash

session 780

strength/skill:
Bench press 3 x 5
superset

bent over rows 3 x 5

WOD: EMOM 18 min

1 - 7 kb swings (20/12) and 7 burpees
2 - 5 kb push press each arm and 7 burpees
3 - 10 jumping lunge and 7 burpees

scale burpees so you get at least 20 sec rest

session 781

strength- c n j

wod- 22/16/10/8/6
c n j (40/30)
lunge

session 782

strength/skill:
O/H squat - find 2RM (20 min)

WOD: amrap 20 min

deadlift x 12 (125/85)
double under x 75
bar muscle up x 5
double under x 75

session 783

strength/skill:
power snatch heavy for day (12 min)
then
3 x 1 @ 90% of above

WOD: 50 sec work / 80 sec rest x 8 rounds

wallball x 12
hang squat clean x 3 @ 70% of 1rm
max pull ups

session 784

strength/skill:
push press - 3 x 3
push jerk - 3 x 2

WOD: amrap 3 min
hspu x 6
TTB x 6

rest 1 min

amrap - 4 min
dip x 8
KTE x 8

rest 1 min

amrap - 3 min
push up x 6
sit up x 6

session 786

strength/skill:
strict press 5 x 5

WOD: for time
50 x KB turkish get up (20/12)
emom 5 swings

session 787

strength/skill:
deadlift - 3 x 2

WOD -
30 x front lunges (50/35)
20 x hang power clean
10 x G2O

15 x KB swings (24/16)
10 x OHS
20 x S2O
30 x goblet squat

session 788

strength/skill:
pull ups 5 x 5 weighted

WOD: 10-1
deadlift (120/85)
DB push jerk (20/15)
pull up

session 789

strength/skill:
dips 5 x 5 weighted

WOD: in pairs
30 min amrap
150 cal bike
150 cal row
100 TTB

1 person working at a time

session 790

strength/skill:
bench press - 7 x 1

WOD: amrap 9 min
burpee box jump x 10
double under x 25
burpee pull up x 10
dpuble under x

session 791

strength/skill:

farmers walk 4 x 10m

WOD: EMOM 21 min
1- single DB squat clean x 10 (20/15)
2- db power snatch x 14
3- 30 sec goblet squat hold

session 792
1rm hang clean

session 793

strength/skill:
snatch balance 5 x 2
or
O/H squat 5 x 2

WOD:
from 0-2min
strict pull up x 8/5
front squat x 2 (70/50)

from 2-4 min
strict pull up x 8/5
front squat x 4

from 4-6 min
strict pull up x 8/5
front squat x 6

continue adding 2 reps to squat until failure

session 794

strength/skill:
find heavy complex of power snatch+full snatch

WOD: for time

75 x sit ups
35 x med ball clean
20 x bar muscle up
35 x med ball clean

75 x sit ups

session   795

strength/skill:
4 x complex
2 strict press+ 4 push press+ 6 push jerk

WOD: AMRAP 12 min
8 x power clean (80/55)
8 x TTB
8 x bar facing burpee

session 796

mash

session 796

strength/skill:
back squat 4 x 10 @60% (perform a set every 2 min)

WOD: 3 rounds

1 min at each station for max reps

box jumps
assault bike
wallball
row
DB push jerk (20/15)
rest 1 min

session 797

strength/skill:
hang power clean find heavy single

WOD: 13 min amrap
1 x devil press
 1 x pull up
 100m run

ascending ladder

session 798

strength/skill:
thruster 3/3/2/2/1/1 (from rack) (perform set every 2:15)

WOD: for time
30 x push press (50/35)
30 x sumo high pull
30 x hspu
200 x double unders
30 x hspu
30 x sumo high pull
30 x push press

session 799

strength/skill:
deadlift - find heavy single (30 min)
or
5 x 5

WOD: 2 min max cals assailt bike

*if time allows
hollow rock or hollow hold tabata

session 800

WOD: 5 rounds for time

32 x wallballs
32 x burpees
32 x lunges with wall ball
32 x KTE
32 x renegade rows without push up (15/7.5)

session 801

750m row @ 85% effort

then
EMOM 7 min - "mini macho man"
3 x power clean (60/40)

3 x front squat
3 x push jerk

5 min rest

EMOM 7 min - "moderate macho man"
3 x power clean (70/45)
3 x front squat
3 x push jerk

rest 5 min

EMOM 7 min - "macho man"
3 x power clean (80/50)
3 x front squat
3 x push jerk

session 802
1rm bs
wod- fuunda 1

session 803

strength/skill:
strict press - 3 x 3
push press - 3 x 3

WOD:

21 x wallballs
7 x muscle up
3 x hang power clean (90/62.5)
15 x wallballs
5 x muscle up
2 x hang power clean
9 x wallballs
3 x muscle up
1 x hang power clean

session 804

strength/skill:

EMOM 12 min

min 1 - 30 sec L- sit
min 2 - 10-30 sec isometric chin up hold

WOD 3 rounds for time

400m run
25 x kb swings (24/16)
200m run
25 x box jumps
100m run
25 x TTB

SESSION 805

strength/skill:
O/H squat- 3 x 10

WOD: 10 - 1

DB power snatch ea arm (20/15)
renegade row

session 806
mash

session 807
strength/skill:
front rack lunges 5 x 10m

WOD: "escape from alcatraz"
in pairs

20 rounds of row or bike
1:00 minute on / :10 sec transition

partner 1 rows on odd minute
partner 2 rows on even minute

set interval timer on machine
work- 1 min
rest - 10 sec

session 808
front squat 5 x 2

15 min amrap
dead/clean/squat/s2o

session 809

strength/skill:
sumo high pull 5 x 3
(perform a set every 90sec)

WOD: "running barbara"

5 rounds for time
20 x pull ups
30 x push ups
40 x sit ups
50 x air squat
400m run

session   810

strength/skill:
1 rm snatch

WOD:
21/15/9
DB cluster (20/15)
burpees

session 811

strength/skill:
back squat 3 x 8

WOD: 5 min amrap
HR push up x 8
O/H db lunge x 16 (20/15)

rest 2 min

amrap 5 min
burpee x 8
wallball x 16

rest 2 min

repeat first amrap

session 812

strength/skill:
deadlift 5 x 5 @ 70 - 75%

WOD: HELEN
3 rounds for time

400m run
21 KB swings (24/16)
12 pull ups

session 813

strength/skill:
4 x complex
2- push press, 2- push jerk with 3 sec pause in dip

WOD: 2 rounds for time
50 x box jumps
30 x dips
30 x DB push press (20/15)
50 x air squats

session 814

strength/skill:
front squat 5 x 3 with tempo 4,4,x,0

WOD:
100 db snatch (20/15)
emom - 2 bar muscle ups (*scaled 2 burpee pull ups)

session 815

strength/skill:
bench press - 5 x 5

WOD: in pairs

100 burpees (partner in prone hold)
100 med ball cleans (partner in squat hold)
100 jumping pull ups (partner in hang)

divide each movement up as need, working partner 1 may only perform reps as
partner 2 is holding position

session 816
power clean
h power clean

wod
sumo chief

session 817

strength/skill:
pulling GVT (ring row, pull up or chin up)
10 sets of 5-10 reps with 3 sec negative.
45 sec rest between sets.

WOD: 10 -1
thrusters (45/32.5)
TTB
KB swing (24/16)

session 818

strength/skill:
overhead squat 3 x 5

WOD: death by wall ball (increase by 2 reps)

rest 3 min

death by burpee (increase by 1 rep)

session 819

strength/skill:

5 x 5 weighted ring dip

WOD amrap 15 min

8 x hang power snatch (40/30)
8 x devils press (20's/15's)
8 x DB hang cleans

session 820
mash

session 821

strength/skill:
O/H lunges 5 x 10m

WOD: 20 min partner
1 person completes a round at a time

10 x alternating dumbell snatches (20/15)
10 x single arm DB overhead box step ups (20inch, 5 each arm)

session 822 dice

session 823
strength/skill:
deadlift 4 x 4

WOD: 2 rounds for time

50 x pull up
40 x lunges (each leg)

30 x power clean (40/30)
20 x shoulder to over head
10 x sdhp

session 823

strength/skill:
hang power clean 5 x 3

WOD: 4 min ladder
kb swing (24/16)
push up
increasing by 2 reps

rest 2 min

4 min ladder
kb snatch
burpee
increasing by 2 reps

rest 2 min

4 min ladder
kb clean + jerk
burpee pull up
increasing by 2 reps

session 824
mash

session 825
strength/skill:
bench press - 3 x 10

WOD: in pairs

running clock

0-2.30
400m run
max partner clap push ups

3.30-6.00
400m run
max partner wall balls

7.00- 9.30
400m run
max partner wall ball sit ups

2 min rest repeat

session 826

strength/skill:
squat clean 4 x 2

wod dice

session 827

strength/skill:
front rack lunges 5 x 10m

WOD:
3 rounds
12 x hang power clean (70/50)
9 x bar facing burpee
6 x turkish get up (24/16) (3 each arm)

session 828

strength/skill:
4 x complex
5 push press, 5 push jerk

WOD: open wod 13.4
AMRAP 7 min
3 clean and jerk (60/40)
3 toes to bar
6 c+j

6 ttb
9 c+j
9 ttb
increase 3 reps untill time is up

rest
if time allows

"durante core workout"
5 rounds for quality
10 hollow rocks
10 v ups
10 tuck up
10 sec hollow hold
1 min rest

session 829

strength/skill:
snatch grip deadlift - 5 x 3

WOD: 7 rounds each for time

200m run
15 x push ups
12 x kb swing (24/16)
9 x air squats
*new round every 3 min
**rx+ new round every 2.30

session 830
mash
21-15-9 reps for time:
Thruster 60/40
Pull-up, strict

3 Rounds for time:
400m run
20 Push-ups
20 Overhead Squats 40/30

30-25-20 reps for time:
GHD Sit-up
Calories, Rower

Rest 5 minutes between workouts

session 831
strength/skill:
DB power snatch 5x 5 each arm

WOD: amrap 20 min

ring row x 12
ring dip x 12
box jump x 12
50m waiter carry right arm (20/15)
50m waiter carry left arm

session 832

strength/skill:
find a heavy front squat single with 3 sec pause

WOD: dice

session 833

strength/skill:
hang snatch 5 x 1

WOD: 10-1
DB thrusters (20/15)
DB hang clean

session 834

strength/skill:
emom 16 min -
min 1 - aim for 10 pull ups
min 2 - aim for 10 ring dips

WOD: open wod 15.3

amrap 14 min
7 x muscle up

50 x wallball
100 x double under

session 835 mash

session 836

strength/skill:
deadball clean

WOD: in pairs
amrap 30 min
back squat (100/70)
200m run every 3min

session 837
dice
1RM front squat

session 834

strength/skill:
bench press 5 x 5

WOD:
dumbbell "DT" (20's/15's)
with 100m waiters walk after each round (50m left arm/ 50m right arm)

session   825

strength/skill:
hang power snatch - 5 x 2

WOD: amrap 14 min

box jump x 60
wallball x 50
KB swing x 40
burpee x 30

session   826

strength/skill:
weighted pull up 5 x 5

WOD:
50 sec on / 80 sec off x 6 rounds

10 x TTB
8 x pull up
max effort cluster (60/40)

rest 2 min

50 sec on / 80 sec off x 4 rounds

10 x dip
10 x push up
max effort S2O (60/40)

session 827
mash

session 828
strength/skill:
5 x max effort ring dips
or
5 x 10 assisted

WOD: 20-1
medball clean
push ups

session 829
strength/skill:
1 cluster every 15 sec for 5 min
rest 2 min
1 cluster every 30 sec for 5 min
rest 2 min
1 cluster every minute for 5 min
(aim is to go heavier each new set)

WOD: 3 rounds for time
DB burpee x 15 (perform burpee on db's then perform a db deadlift instead of jumping)
DB push jerk x 10 (20's,15's)

session 830
strength/skill:
deadlift - 5 x 5

WOD: amrap 12 min
15 x box jump
12 x push press (50/35)
9 x TTB

session 831
mash

session 832
strength/skill:
sumo high pull - 5 x 3

session 833
open wod 17.1

session 834

strength/skill:
bench press - 5 x 3

WOD:
amrap- 5 min
8 x pull ups
25 double unders

1 min rest

amrap 5 min
8 x TTB
25 x double under

session 835
strength
back squat 5 x 5

wod: 5 rft

100m run
12 wallball
100m run
12 sit up

session 836

strength
power clean and jerk 3/3/2/1/1

wod
8 min ladder
c+j (70/50)
10 air squats

session 848

strength/skill:
front squat 4 x 4 (2@ 4.2.x.0/ 2@ 1.0.x.0)
front squat 3 x 8 (1 and 1/4)

WOD: amrap 8 min
burpee muscle ups

session 849
17.4

session 850

strength/skill:
10 min to find 3rm push press
then 3 x 3 at 90% of 3rm

WOD: 4 rounds for time

15 x front squat (60/40) (*no rack)
10 x hang power clean
15 x bar over burpees
rest 90 sec

session 851

strength - 3 pos clean

wod - 6 rounds 12 db snatch 20 push up

session 852

strength/skill:
bench press waves - 5/3/1
or 5 x 5 for beginners

WOD: for time
40 kb swings (24/16)
30 cal assault bike
20 jumping lunges

session 853

mash

1 mile run
"isabel" (50/35)
1 mile run
"grace"
1 mile run
"elizabeth"

*elizabeth is squat cleans

session 854

strength/skill:
dip support 5 x max effort
chin over bar hold 5 x max effort

WOD: amrap 20 min
12 x wallball
400m run
12 x burpee box jump
400m run
12 x pull up
400m run

session 855

open wod 17.5

session 856

strength/skill:
back squat 7 x 2

WOD: 1 min assault bike for cal

session 857
strength/skill:
find heavy complex of-
squat clean/4 x walking lunge/cluster/4 x walking lunge/squat clean

WOD: for time
50 clean and jerks (40/30)
emom - 4 burpees

session 858
dice

session 859

strength/skill:
weighted dips 5 x 5

WOD: for time

100 x air squat
80 x push jerk (30/25)
60 x wallball
40 x push press
20 x thruster

session 860

strength/skill:
power snatch - 3/3/2/2/1/1

WOD: 13 min ladder (ascending 1 rep)
devil press (20/15)
jumping lunge each leg
30 double unders each

session 861

strength/skill:
weighted pull ups 5 x 5

WOD: 3 rounds
6 x clean and jerk (60/40)
12 x strict pull ups
24 x TTB
48 x box jumps

session 862
dice

session 863

strength/skill:
push press 3 x 5
push jerk 3 x 3

wod:

75 DB hang clean and jerk
4 burpees emom

session 864

strength/skill:

L-sit hang from bar - accumulate 5 min

WOD:
10-1 - deadlift (110/75)
20-2 pull up (20,18,16,14,12etc…)

session 865

strength/skill:
3rm thruster (may use rack)

WOD: 20 min ascending ladder
cluster (40/30)
hang power clean
s2o

*do 1 cluster, 1 hang power clean then 1s20,
then 2 x clusters, 2 x hang power clean, 2 x s2o,
then 3 x cluster, 3 x hang power clean , 3 x s2o. etc……
*every time you need rest or let go of the bar perform 10 burpees

session 866

strength/skill:
back squat waves - 3/2/1/3/2/1

WOD:
21/15/9

DB snatch (22.5/15) (reps each arm)
TTB
wallball

session 867

strength/skill:
overhead squat - 6/6/4/4/2/2

WOD:
12 x muscle ups
3 x clean and jerk (100/70)
9 x muscle ups

2 x c+j
6 x muscle ups
1 x c+j

*scaled - double amount of burpee pull-ups
clean and jerk should be a heavy but not max effort weight

session 868
strength/skill:
snatch deadlift - 5 x 5

WOD: 2 rounds for time

30 x push up
200m run
30 x deadlift (40/30)
100m sprint
30 x push press
200m run

session 870   28/4/17
mash

session 871
in pairs
amrap 15 min
partner A runs 400m
partner B does turkish get ups (15/7.5)
score is number of get ups

rest 5 min

amrap 30

50 wall balls (partner A does cleans, partner B holds air squat. Air squat must be held for reps to count)
50 push ups (partner A does push up, partner B holds plank)
50 sit ups (partner A does sit up, partner B holds L-sit)
50 x DB snatches (partner A does snatches, partner B olds plate over head)
rest 5 min

amrap 5 min
one for one burpees

session 872
back squat

dice

session 873
strength/skill:
4 x complex - 3+2 push press/push jerk

WOD:
9/15/21/27
burpees
kb swing (24/16)
db push jerk left arm (22.5/15)
db push jerk right arm

session 874

strength/skill:
deadlift - 15 min to find a heavy a heavy double
 4 min rest
then 5 x 3 @ 70% of 2rm (speed reps, 90 secs rest)

WOD: 3 rounds for time

DB box step up x 18 (22.5/15)
DB hang squat clean x 12

session 875
strength/skill:
bench press 5 x 5

WOD: for time
15 x clean and jerk (50/35)
3 rounds

session 876
mash

session 877

strength/skill:
db snatch 5 x 3 each arm

WOD: amrap 30min
as partners (1 working at a time)

20 thrusters (50/35)
20 burpee box jumps

30 thrusters (40/30)
30 burpee box jumps

40 thrusters (30/20)
40 burpee box jumps

50 thrusters (20/15)
50 burpee box jumps

max distance on bike/rower in remaining

session 879

strength/skill:
4 x complex- power snatch/ 2xO-H squat/ snatch

WOD: for time

30 X hang power clean (42.5/30)
9 X burpee muscle up (*scale 18 burpee pull up)
30 X push press
7 X burpee muscle up (*14 burpee pull ups)
30 X thrusters
5 X burpee muscle ups (*10 burpee pull ups)
30 X bar over burpees
3 X burpee muscle ups (*6 burpee pull ups

session 880

strength/skill:
back squat 6x3 @ 88-90%

WOD: 3 rounds
single arm DB cluster x 16 (alternating 22.5/15)
sit ups x 40

session 881
mash

session 884

strength/skill:
sumo high pull 5 x 3

WOD:
60 x double under
20 x wallball
15 x deadlift (100/70)
90 x double under
20 x wallball
15 x deadlift
120 x double under
20 x wallball
15 x deadlift

session 885
strength/skill:
power clean - 3/2/1/2/3

WOD:
AMRAP 15 min
kb swing x 40 (24/12)
clean and jerk x 30 (50/35)
box jump x 20

session 886

strength/skill:
strict press - 5 x 3

WOD: 12 min running clock
amrap 3 min- db snatch (22.5/15)
amrap 3 min- burpee pull up

amrap 2 min- db snatch
amrap 2 min- burpee pull up
amrap 1 min- db snatch
amrap 1 min- burpee pull up

session 887

mash

9/15/21
kb swing
thruster (35/25)
pull up

rest

5 rounds
50 double under
5 squat clean (70/50)

session 888
strength/skill:
DB push press 5 x 5 each arm

WOD: E2MOM for 20 min (10 rounds)
1 round of cindy
100m sprint (run hard)

session 889

back squat 5 x 3 (aim is working 85% through to 88% +2.5kgs)

WOD: dice

session 890
strength/skill:
ring dips 5 x 5 weighted (or 5 x 10 banded)

WOD: 17ML.3
3 rounds for time
18 HSPU

15 Hang squat clean (70/50)

session 891

strength/skill:
O/H squat 3 x 3

WOD: amrap 25 min

Wall balls x 35
single arm o/h DB lunges x 70 (22.5/15) (35 each arm)
double under x 100

session 892

strength/skill:
Bench press 3 x 5
superset
bent over rows 3 x 5

wod:
run 400 m
4 x bear complex (50/35)
run 300 m
3 x bear complex
run 200 m
2x bear complex
run 100m
1 x bear complex

session 893

Monster Mash

3 Rounds for time:
800m run
8 Deadlifts 165/115

21-15-9:
Overhead Squat 50/35
*5 Ring MU's after each round

*Rest 10 minutes after each round

session   894

partner wod: amrap 40min
air squat x 30
KB swing x 20 (24/16)
burpee x 10

1 partner completes a round wile the other rests

starting on "0" and every 10 min mark, both partners run 400m

session 895

strength/skill:
bench press 5 x 5

WOD: 5 rounds

1 min sumo high pull (30/25)
1 min push press
1 min double unders
1 min rest

session 898   1

WOD: partner wod.

20 min ascending ladder. (ascending by 2)

burpee box step up

200m run

divide reps as needed

session 902

strength/skill:
push press- waves 5/3/5/3/5/3

WOD: AMRAP 12 min
push up x 15
power clean x 10 (60/40)
cluster x 5

session   903

strength/skill:
hang squat clean - 3 x 3

WOD: amrap 20 min

double under x 50
DB man makers x 20 (22.5/15)
double under x 50
DB snatch x 20

session 904

strength/skill:
deadlift - 10/8/6/4/2 (AHAP with max 120 sec rest between sets)

WOD: 3 rounds
14 x kb swing (24/16)
7 x muscle up (10 burpee pull ups for scaled)

straight into

3 rounds
21 x wall ball
21 x TTB

straight into

200m DB farmers carry (choose own load)

session 905

partner amrap - 20 min

60 x partner wallballs
60 x DB box step ups

rest 10 min

partner amrap - 15 min
20 x turkish get up (15/7.5)
20 x burpee pull up

(break up as needed)

session 906
dice

session 907
strength/skill:
bench press - 10/8/6/4/2/2/2

WOD: "fran"
21/15/9
thrusters (42.5/30)
pull ups

session 909

strength/skill:
4 x complex - 5 front squat/ 3 push press

WOD: amrap 3 min
deadlift x 2 (140/100)
bar over burpee x 4

rest 2 min

amrap 5 min
deadlift x 4 (100/70)
bar over burpee x 8

rest 2 min

amrap 7 min
sumo high pull x 6 (60/40)
bar over burpee x 12

session 910

mash

4 rounds
400m run
15 x wallballs
15 x pull ups

rest

2 rounds
30 x push press
400 m farmer carry (22.5/15)
20 x TTB

session 911

partner amrap 40 min
50 x plate snatches (20/15)(partner holds plate over head)

40 x pull ups (partner hangs)

30 x man makers (22.5/15)(partner holds DB's in rack)

200 m odd object carry (heavy d-ball/heavy KB/box jump/heavy DB)

100 x one for one buprees

session 912   12/7/17

strength/skill:
snatch balance - 5 x 2

WOD: 3 x 5 min amraps

hspu x 5
deadlift x 7 (80/55)
TTB x 9

rest 2 min

session 914

strength/skill:
bench press - 5 x 5

WOD: for time
20 x burpee
30 x db push press left arm (22.5/15)
30 x db push press right arm
30 x racked db squat (left arm)
30 x racked db squat (right arm)
30 x db snatch left arm
30 x db snatch right arm
20 x burpee

session 915

strength/skill:
strict press 5 x 3

WOD: amrap 12 min

9 x DB deadlift (22.5/15)
6 x burpee
3 DB power clean

Friday Mash: 916

2 Rounds for time:
22 Thrusters (40/30)
22 Pull-ups

2 Rounds for time:
22 Deadlifts (100/70)
22 hspu

2 Rounds for time:
22 Toes-to-bar
22 Hang Power Snatch (50/35)

*Rest 5 minutes between workouts

session 919

strength/skill:
overhead squat - 4 x 6 @75%

WOD:
5 rounds each for time
10 x push press (40/30)
12 x burpee
15 x kb swing (24/16)
rest 90 sec

(each rounds is an all out effort, no pacing or holding back)

session 920

40 min partner amrap

75 x pull ups
75 x front rack lunge (40/30)
6 x 200m sprints (3 each)
75 x back squat
75 x push ups

(one partner working at a time, swap every minute on the minute

session 921
mash

session 922

strength/skill:
front rack lunge 5 x 10m

WOD: 21/15/9
box jump
hspu

rest 2 min

15/9/6
box jump
db thrusters (22.5/15)

rest 2 min

9/6/3
burpee box jump
muscle up

session   923

strength/skill:
bench press 4 x 8
super set
push press (from ground)

WOD: 20 min clock

1.6 km run
then in remainder time
ascending ladder

2 x strict pull ups
2 x man makers

4 x strict pull ups
4 x man makers

etc……

session   924

strength/skill:
back squat 4 x 7 all sets @ 75%

WOD: 4 rounds starting a new round every 5 min
max effort hang power cleans (60/40)
max effort wall balls
max effort TTB
max effort double unders

once a movement is broken you must move to the next.

session 925

strength/skill:
strict press - 5 x 5

WOD: 6 rounds for time
cluster x 4 (60/40)
burpee x 8
deadlift x 12

session 926
strength/skill:
EMOM: 5 min
power clean/ 2 x front squat

EMOM: 5 min
hang squat clean/ front squat

EMOM: 5 min
full clean

rest 2 min between each emom.

WOD: for time
50 x power clean (60/40)
emom - death by pull up (starting at 5 pull ups increasing by 1 pull up each
minute)

session 927

strength/skill:
push ups on rings 5 x 10

WOD: 4 rounds

75 x double under
15 x kb snatch right arm (24/16)
15 x kb snatch left arm

session 929

strength/skill:

bench press- 4 x 7 ahap

WOD: amrap 17 min

100 x TTB
50 x air squat
25 x clean and jerk (50/35)

session 930

strength/skill:
ring dips - 5 x max effort

WOD: 10 rounds
12 x O/H db lunge (22.5/15) (6 each arm)
6 x over db burpees

session 931

mash

amrap 9 min
9 x deadlift (80/55)
9 x chest to bar
9 x KTE

rest

amrap 10 min
35 x double unders
5 x hand release push ups
10 x push press (50/35)

rest

if time allows

27/21/15/9
sit ups
wallballs

session 932

WOD: partner wod

30 min running clock

partner 1 runs 200m with med ball
partner 2 performs amrap of thrusters   (30/20)

partner 1 skips 150 skips
partner 2 performs amrap of kb snatch (24/16)

partner 1 runs 200m with med ball
partner 2 performs amrap of pullups/ring rows

partner 1 skips 150 skips
partner 2 performs amrap of wall balls

go back to start and swap roles

session 933
sod dice back squat 5x5 80%

session   934

strength/skill:
power clean/ push press/ split jerk - find heavy

WOD: 10-1
renegade rows (22.5/15) (1 rep is - push up/ row right arm, push up row left arm)
db hang power clean

sesssion   935

strength/skill: deadlift - 4 x 3 @ 80%

WOD: amrap 8min
15 x kb swing (24/16)
10 x o/h KB lunge left arm
15 x KB swing
10 x o/h KB lunge right arm

rest 3 min

50 KB swing for time

session 936
strength/skill:
bench press 5 x 5

WOD: 25 rounds
1 x power clean (85/60)
3 x TTB
5 x lateral bar hops

session 937

mash

18/15/12/9
deadball clean (open weight)
muscle up (1/3 reps) (*scale burpee pull ups)

rest

4 rounds
30 sit ups
5 x push jerks (80/55)

session 942

partner wod

for time:

5km row or 250/175 cal assault bike
60 x wall ball
60 x box jump

wile partner A is working, partner B is holding plank. Once plank is broken,

session 949

strength/skill:
bench press - 5 x 3

WOD: 10-1
DB burpee deadlifts (22.5/15)
DB push jerks

session 950

strength/skill:
weighted dips - 5 x 5

WOD:
7 rounds for time
35 x double under
7 x hspu
5 x cluster (60/40)

session 951

strength/skill:
overhead squat 5 x 5

WOD: for time

15 x TTB
50 x O/H squat (30/20)
15 x TTB
50 x thruster
15 x TTB
50 x box jump
15 x TTB

session 952

b squat 92 x2 94x1 90x 3

session   953

strength/skill:
power clean - 3/3/2/2

WOD: 1/2/3/4/5/4/3/2/1
muscle up
clean and jerk (70/50)

(scale burpee pull up x2)

session   954

strength/skill:
deadlift 3 x 2 AHAP

WOD: amrap 12 min
18 x alternating one arm DB cluster (22.5/15)
9 x TTB

session 956

partner amrap 40 min

10 x med ball clean
10 x sit up
10 x kb swing (24/16)
10 x renegade rows (22.5/15)
200m run

add 5 reps to everything each round
break reps up as needed

session 958

session 959
strength/skill:
push press 5 x 5

WOD: for time
40 x burpee box overs
40 x box jumps
40 x burpees
40 x box step ups with DB's

emom - 4 x DB hang power clean (22.5/15)

session 959
dice

session 960

strength/skill:
l-sit, accumulate 3 min

WOD:
with 25 min cap
run 1.6 km

then

get as far through open workout 14.5 as possible

21/18/15/12/9/6/3
thrusters
bar over burpees

session   961

strength/skill:
bench press 1rm

WOD: 17 min ladder

1 x power clean (80/55)
1 x shuttle run (door to driveway foot path)
8 x push up

8 x Toes to bar

2 x power clean
2 x shuttle run
8 x push up
8 x TTB

3 x power clean
3 x shuttle run
8 x push up
8 x TTB

ETC……

(power cleans and shuttle run increase a rep each round, push up and TTB
remain at 8 reps)

session 962

strength/skill:
hang squat clean - 4 x 3

WOD: for time

40 x s2o (50/35)
20 x pullup
5 x rope climb

20 x s2o
10 x pull up
3 x rope climb

session 963

amrap 30

50 wall balls (partner A does cleans, partner B holds air squat. Air squat must be
held for reps to count)
50 push ups (partner A does push up, partner B holds plank)
50 sit ups (partner A does sit up, partner B holds L-sit)
50 x DB snatches (partner A does snatches, partner B olds plate over head)
rest 5 min

amrap 5 min
one for one burpees

session 965
strength/skill:
overhead squat - 5 x 5

WOD: amrap 9 min
8 x push press (40/30)
12 x C2B
100m sprint

rest 3 min

tabata - TTB

session 966

strength/skill:
sumo high pull 5 x 5

WOD: "fight gone bad"

 3 rounds
1 min of each

wallball
sumo high pull (35/30)
box jump
push press
row
rest 1 min

session 968

40 min partner amrap

75 x burpee pull up
75 x goblet lunges (24/16)
800 m run
75 x partner sit ups (with wall ball)
75 x partner wall balls

sessio 970

session 973

40 min partner amrap

100 x O/H single arm db lunges (22.5/15)
100 x db snatch
100 x single arm db clusters

wile partner "1" works partner "2" rows or bikes 15/12 cals then swap

score is reps and cals combined

session   975

strength/skill:
clean and jerk 4 x 2

WOD:

21 x hspu
5 x clean and jerk (90/62.5)
15 x hspu
4 x c n j
9 x hspu
3 x c n j

session 982

strength/skill:
bench press - 5 x 7

WOD:
50/40/30/20/10

double under
sit ups

12 x db snatch after each round

Session 983

strength/skill:
O/H squat - 5 x 5

WOD: 20 min ascending ladder

burpee box step up
power snatch (40/30)
200m run

Session 984
Strength/skill:
Deadlift - 3 x 5 @ 65%

WOD: 3 min window
24 x wallball
12 x single DB box step ups
Max effort cluster (60/40)

Rest 1 min
Repeat x 4 rounds

985
Strength:
Strict press - 5/3/1/5/3/1

WOD: amrap 7 min
40 x double unders
12 x Db push press

Rest 3 min

Amrap 5 min
30 x double unders
6 x renegade row *no push up

Strength:

Front squat -
20 reps
1 minute rest
10 reps
30 sec rest
5 reps
30 sec rest
5 reps

WOD: for time
30 x sumo high pull (20/15)
30 x front squat
30 x hang squat clean
30 x power snatch
30 x overhead squat

Emom - 5 x burpees

Session 986

Strength-
Deadlift 5 x 5

WOD: 21/15/9
Back squat (60/40)
Push jerk
*2 x man maker after each round

Session 987

Strength:
Clean and jerk - find 2rm

WOD: amrap 20 min
50 x sit up
30 x Db snatch
50 x burpee
30 x single Db clean and jerk

Session 988

Strength endurance:
Accumulate 100 push ups in as little sets as possible.

WOD: for time
1.6km farmer carry
Every time you have to break perform 5 thrusters.

Session 989
Strength:
Bent over row- 7/7/5/5/3/3

WOD: 5 rounds for time
15 x push jerk (50/35)
15 x hang power clean
40 x double unders

Session 990
Strength:

Front squat -
20 reps
1 minute rest
10 reps
30 sec rest
5 reps
30 sec rest
5 reps

WOD: amrap 12 min
35 x medball clean
8 x devil press

Session 991
For time

1 round
150 x double unders
30 x high pull (40/30)
30 x burpees

Into
2 rounds
75 x double unders
15 x sumo high pull
15 x burpee
Into
3 rounds
50 x double unders
10 x sumo high pull
10 x burpee

Session 992
Strength-
Strict press - 7/7/5/5/3/3

WOD:
5 x 3 min amraps

2 x renegade row
4x power clean (40/30)
6 x sit up

Rest 1 min Between amraps

Session 993

Strength:
bent over row 5 x 5

WOD: for time
300 x walking lunge
EMOM - 5 x wallball

Session 994
For time

1.6km run
Into
3 rounds
30 x Db snatch

30 x sit up
30 x strict press (30/20)
Into
1.6k run

Session 995

Strength:
Hang squat clean - 5x3 *touch and go

WOD: running clock
EMOM x 5 min
5 x thruster (20/15)
5 x burpee
Strait into
EMOM X 5 min
7 x thruster
7 x burpee
Strait into
EMOM X 5 min
9 x thruster
9 x burpee

Session 996
Front squat -
20 reps
1 minute rest
10 reps
30 sec rest
5 reps
30 sec rest
5 reps

WOD: for time
30 x Turkish get up
Emom - 7 x KB swings

Session 997

20 rounds for time

1 x deadlift (120/85)
5 x bar over burpees
15 x double unders

Accessories:
Hollow rock -
30 seconds on 30 seconds off x 7

Session 998
Strength- work up to a power clean 2rm. Then do 3 further sets of 2 at 90% of 2rm

WOD:
50 x sit ups
50 x push ups
50 x sit ups
50 x squats
50 x sit ups
50 x lunges
50 x sit ups

Session 999

Strength-
bent over row - 7 x 3

WOD: ascending 12 min ladder
1 x renegade row
1 x double Db snatch

2 x renegade row
2 x double Db snatch

3 x renegade row
3 x double Db snatch

Etc.........

Session 1000
Strength-
Push press 5x5

WOD: 5 rounds for time
30 x wallball
5 x cluster (70/47.5)

Session 1001

3 rounds For time
800m run
15 x deadlift (100/70)
15 x Db push press

Accessories:
Hollow rocks - accumulate 75
Plank - accumulate 5 min

Session 1002
Strength-
bent over rows 5x5
After last set drop weight and do 1 set of 20

WOD:
21/15/9
Thruster (30/20)
Push up

Rest 3 min

15/12/9
Thruster (40/30)
Bar over burpee

Rest 3 min

9/6/3
Thruster (60/40)
Renegade row

Session 1003

Strength -
Work up to 80-85% of your clean and jerk

Then set a clock for 30 min and perform 1 clean and jerk every minute on the minute.

Session 1004
For time:

100 x double unders
30 x hang power snatch (40/30)
8 x Turkish gets ups

75 x double unders
20 x hang power snatch
6 x Turkish get up

50 x double unders
10 x hang power snatch
4 x Turkish get up

25 x double unders
5 x hang power snatch
2 x Turkish get up

Session 1005
Strength -
Deadlift - 3x5

WOD:
For time
50 x thruster (50/35)
50 x Db snatch
*emom 5 x burpees

Session 1006
Skill: 20 min of handstand practice

WOD: run bike or row for 30 min

Session 1007

Strength-
Strict press 7 x 3

WOD: 21/15/9
Push press (50/35)
Hang power clean
Push up

Session 1008

Strength
Bent over row 5x5

WOD: 3 min window
30 x wallball
10 x Db snatch
Max effort jumping lunge

Rest 1 min repeat x 6 rounds

Session 1009
For time:

20 x clean and jerk (60/40)
50 x bar facing burpee
20 x clean and jerk

Accessories:
Hollow rocks 5 x 15
Plank 3 x 1-2 min

Session 1010
Strength:
Deadlift- 3 x 5

WOD: amrap 12 min
18 x Kb sumo high pull
100m sprint

18 x Kb snatch
100m sprint

Session 1011

Strength-
Squat clean + 4 front squats
5 sets

WOD: 3 rounds for time
8 x Db hang power clean
10 x Db push press
12 x lunge with racked dbs

Accessories-
3 x max effort banana split

Session 1012

Strength -
Strict press 5 x 3
Bent over row 5 x 3

WOD:
30/20/10
kB swing
Sit ups

Rest 2 min

10/20/30
kB swing
Push up

Session 1013
For time
65 x wallball
75 x double under
10 x front squat (80/55)
800 m run
10 x front squat

65 x double under
75 x wallball

Session 1014

Strength-
clean and jerk 1rm

E3mom x 5 rounds - 1 clean and jerk @ 90% of above 1rm

WOD: amrap 15 min
75 x hang power clean (30/20)
50 x push press
25 x hang power snatch
*emom - 4 burpees

Session 1015
Strength- hang power clean 2rm

WOD-
21 x deadlift (100/70)
3 x Turkish get up
15 x deadlift
5 x Turkish get up
9 x deadlift
7 x Turkish get up

Session 1016

Strength
Bent over row 5 x 5
And/or
Pull ups (if possible)

WOD: for time
50 x overhead plate lunge (20/15)
10 x renegade row
40 x O/h lunge
8 x renegade row
30 x O/h plate lunge

6 x renegade row
20 x O/h plate lunge
4x renegade row
10 x O/h plate lunge
2 x renegade row

Session 1017

5 rft
5 x power clean (60/40)
10 x front squat
5 x push jerk
15 x burpee

Rest 90 sec between rounds

Session 1018

Strength
Power snatch - 5 x 2

WOD:
30 x double Db clean and jerk

3 min rest

50 push-ups for time

2 min rest

30 x Double Db hang snatch

Session 1019
15-1
Wallball
Sit up
*1 x bear complex after every round

Session 1020

Strength/skill:
Deadlift 3x5

WOD: Emom (every minute on the minute)
1 x Db deadlift
1 x Db hang power clean
20 x double under

*increase Db movements x 1 each minute.
Continue in this fashion untill you can't beat the clock.

Session 1021

Strength
Bent over row - 5 x 5

30/20/10
Front rack lunge (50/35)
Single arm push press

Session 2022
2 min window
200m sprint
15 x sir squat
Max effort cluster in remainder (50/35)

Rest 1 min
Repeat x 5 rounds

Session 1023

3 rounds for time
12 x hang power clean (60/40)
12 x devils press

Rest

20 Turkish get ups for time

Session 1024
Strength
Sumo high pull - 5 x 5

WOD:
5 rounds for time
400m run with wallball
200m farmer carry

Session 1025

Amrap 16 min

50 x Db hang snatch
100 x jumping lunge
150 x bar over burpees

*every 2 minutes on the minute perform 4 x deadlifts @ (100/70)

Session 1026

Strength/
20 min to work up to a power clean and strict press

WOD: 3 rounds for time
12 x barbell hang squat clean (60/40)
15 x Db push jerk

Rest 5 min

For time
100 x sit ups
Emom - 15 second plank

Session 1027

Amrap 9 min
12 x Db snatch
24 x push up

Rest 3 min

Into

3 rounds for time
15 x kB swing
15 x burpee

Session 1028
Strength/skill:
Back squat 5 x 5 @80%
Split squat 3 x 10 w/dbs

WOD: amrap 7 min
8 x Box jump
8 x hang power clean (50/35)
8 x ttb

Session 1029
20 min partner amrap
Partner A - 400m run
Partner B -
12 x kB lunge
6 x deadball over shoulder
12 x kB push jerk

Rest 5 min

Amrap 10min
Partner A - 100m farmer carry
Partner B -
8 x burpee
16 x wallball

Session 1030

5 rounds for time
12 x hspu
6 x power clean (70/47.5)

Rest

4 rounds for time
25 x sit up
15 x kB swing

5 x ring muscle up

Session 1031
Strength/skill:
Bench press - 5 x 3

WOD: 3 rounds for time
12 x Db cluster (22.5/15)
12 x renegade row
*1 min rest between rounds

Session 1032
Strength/skill:
Turkish get up - 15 min to find a heavy

WOD: for time
50 x Db snatch (22.5/15)
30 x burpee box jump
10 x single Db box step up
800m run
10 x single Db step up
30 x burpee box jump
50 x Db snatch

Session 1033
Strength/skill:
Hang squat clean/ hang power clean - 5 x 1 + 2

WOD: amrap 12 min
1 x Clean and jerk (50/35)
5 x pull up
10 x push up

*increase c+j x 1 each round

Session 1034

Strength/skill:
Back squat - 3 x 5 @ 70%*
Split squat - 3 x 10 unweighted
*deload - don't go heavier wade

WOD: 3 rounds for time
15 x thruster (40/30)
15 x ttb
400m run

Session 1035

Strongman

WOD: amrap 8 min
8 x Db hang clean and jerk
6 x wallball
4 x burpee pull up

Session 1036

21 x hspu
5 x rope climb
15 x hspu
3 x rope climb
9 x hspu
1 x rope climb

Rest

12 min ascending ladder
10 x air squat
10 x push up
1 x power snatch (50/35)

Increase squat and push ups x 2
Snatch remains @ 1

Session 1037

Strength/skill:
Pull up - 4 x max effort sets
Or

Accumulate 10-15 slow negative reps

WOD: 5 rounds for time
60 x double unders
5 x deadlift(60/40)
4 x hang power clean
3 x front squat
2 x push press
1 x push jerk

Rest 1 min

Session 1038

Strength/skill:
Strict press - 5 x 5

WOD: 21/15/9/15/21
Burpee
Kte

Session 1039

Strength/skill:
Back squat 4 x 8 @75%
Bulgarian split squat - 3 x 8 w/dbs

WOD:
amrap 8 min of Wallballs
Emom - 8 x box jump

Session 1040

40 min amrap

Partner WOD

40 x cal bike or row
30 x synchro bar facing burpees
20 x synchro TTB
10 x partner deadlifts
200m partner farmer carry (22.5/16)

Session 1041

2 rounds for time
20 x wallball
10 x power snatch (40/30)
20 x wallball
10 x clean and jerk
20 x wallball
10 x overhead squat
20 x wallball
10 x hang power clean

Session 1042

Strength/skill:
Sumo high pull - 5 x 3

WOD: 3 min window
20 x air squat
20 x push up
20 x sit up
Max effort Single Db hang clean & jerk (22.5/15
*if fail to get to Db reduce all reps x 5 h

Session 1043

Strength/skill:
Pendlay row - 5 x 3

WOD: 20 min ascending ladder
2 x renegade row *no push up (22.5/15)
2 x ttb
Increase x 2
*every 4 min perform 4 x Turkish get up

Session 1044

Strength/skill:
Close grip Bench press - 5 x 5

WOD: 8 rounds for time
30 x double unders
8 x push press (40/30)
3 x bar muscle up

Session 1045

Strength
Back squat 3 x 10 @70%
Split squat 3 x 15 each leg

WOD: amrap 10 min
20 x O/h single DB lunge (22.5/15)
5 x hang power clean (70/47.5)
10 x bar facing burpees

Session 1046

40min strongman

WOD: amrap 8 min
1 x deadball over bar
1 x man maker
*increase deadball x 1 each round

Session 1047

3 rounds for time
50 x double unders
15 x front squat (50/35)
9 x hspu

Rest

Amrap 15 min
10 x burpee to target
12 x Db* front rack box step over (22.5/15)
2 x rope climb
*1 DB

Session 1048

Strength/skill:
Power clean + hang power clean
Work to heavy

WOD: amrap 12 min
8 x pull up
12 x box jump
1 x deadlift (140/100)
*increase deadlift x 1 each round

Session 1049

Strength/skill:
Elevated feet ring rows 5 x 10-15

WOD: for time
50/40/30/20/10
kB swing (24/16)
Sit up
*100m front rack carry after each round

Session 1050

Strength/skill:
Hang power snatch - 5 x 2

WOD: 3 rounds for time
12 x double DB Hang snatch (22.5/15)
12 x burpee over DB
400m run

Session 1051
Strength
Back squat 4x8 @ 70%
Bulgarian split squat 3 x 12 each leg

WOD: amrap 10 min
30 x wallball
1 x clean and jerk (80/55)
*increase c&j x 1 each round

Session 1052
Amrap 20 min
Partner 1- 20/15 cals
Partner 2 - amrap of Cindy

Rest 10 min

Amrap 20 min
Partner 1 - 20/15 cals
Partner 2 - amrap
5 x Db thruster, 5 x ttb, 5 x renegade row

Session 1053

Amrap 13 min
25 x deadlift (100/70)
25 x wallball
25 x hspu

Rest

3 rounds for time
50 x double under
15 x knees to elbow

15 x push jerk (50/35)

Session 1054
Strength/skill:
Accumulate 3 min in l-sit
Accumulate 3 min in at top of dip

WOD: amrap 25 min
800m run
200m overhead plate carry (20/15)
100m farmer carry (22.5/15)
30 x box jump

Session 1055
Strength/skill:
Pendlay row - 4 x 6 (3 sec eccentric)

WOD: for time
30 x man maker (50/35)
Every break perform 2 x Turkish get up (22.5/15)

Session 1056
Strength/skill:
Push press + push jerk 5 x (2+3)

WOD: for time
100 x doburpeeuble unders
40 x burpee pull up
20 x clean and jerk (60/40)

Session 1057
Strength/skill:
Back squat - 3 x 10 @60%
Bulgarian split squat - 3 x 10 each leg (no weight)

WOD: amrap 8 min

30 x wallball
20 x ttb
10 x Db snatch (22.5/15)

Session 1058
40 min strongman

WOD: amrap 8 min
12 x alternating DB Clean and jerk
18 x sit up

Session 1059
3 rounds for time
15 x power snatch (40/30)
10 x bar facing burpees

Rest

3 rounds for time
21 x thruster (40/30)
15 x hang power clean
9 x hspu

Session 1060
Strength/skill:
Back rack lunges- 4 x 6 each leg

WOD: amrap 8 min
8 x Db box step overs (22.5/15)
12 x pull up

Rest 3 min

Amrap 5 min
3 x Sumo high pull 60/40
6 x box jump
9 x late bar hops

Session 1061

Strength/skill:
Ring dips - 10/10/8/8/6/6
*add weight to achieve reps

WOD: 5 rounds for time
25 x wallball
50 x double under
25 x kB swing (24/16)
*rest 1 min after each round

Session 1062
Strength/skill:
Bench press- 3 rm then
2x2 @95% of above

WOD: amrap 12 min
100m run
10 x TTB
100m run
10 x push ups

Session 1063
Strength
Deadlift - work to 3rm then 2 x 2 @ 95% of above weight

WOD: for time
8 x devil press (22.5/15)
5 x squat clean (60/40)

8 x devil press
4 x squat clean (70/45)

8 x devil press
3 x squat clean (80/55)

8 x devil press
2 x squat clean (90/60)

8 x devil press
1 x squat clean (100/65)

Session 1064

Partner amrap 40 min
400m kB carry (24/16)
100 x wallball
400m kB carry
100 x wallball sit ups
400m carry
Amrap 1 for 1 burpees in remainder

Session 1065

15/12/9
Push jerk (50/35)
Bar facing burpee

Rest

15/12/9
Box jump
Bar facing burpee

Rest

15/12/9
Db hang power clean
Bar facing burpee

Session 1066
Strength/skill:
Weighted negative pull ups - accumulate 10-15 reps

WOD: 3 rounds for time
15 x pull up
20 x kB swing (24/16)
800m run

Session 1067
Strength/skill:
Hang squat clean/squat clean - work to heavy

WOD: 2 min window
25 x wallball

30 x double unders
Max hang squat clean (60/40)

Rest 2 min
Repeat x 5 rounds
*if fail to get to cleans drop reps x 5

Session 1068
Strength/skill:
Hang power snatch/ power snatch - work to heavy

WOD: 3 rounds for time
30 x KTE
10 x Turkish get up (15/10)

Session 1069

Strength/skill:
Deadlift - 2 x 3 @last weeks top weight

WOD: amrap 18 min
8 x Db snatch (22.5/15)
8 x burpee
1 x bear complex (40/30)

*increase bear complex x 1 each round

Session 1070

40 min strongman

WOD: amrap 8 min
1 x left arm DB thruster
1 x right arm thruster
5 x pull up
*increase thrusters x 1 rep each round

Session 1071

5 Rounds for time
26 x walking lunges
5 x bar muscle ups

Rest

4 rounds for time
12 x front squat (60/40) *no rack
50 x double unders

Session 1072

Strength/skill:
Front - squat 1 & 1/4's
3 x 3

WOD: for time
200m O/H plate carry (20/15)
15 x hang power clean (40/30)
200m FARMER carry (22.5/15)
10 x hang power clean (60/40)
200m FARMER carry
5 x hang power clean (80/55)
200m O/H plate carry

Session 1073

Strength/skill:
Bench press 5 x 5

WOD: 2 rounds for time
15 x renegade row (22.5/15)
20 x left arm Db push jerk
15 x renegade row
20 x right arm Db push jerk

Session 1074

Deadlift- 5x5

WOD: amrap 12 min
200m run
14 x box jump
200m run
7 x burpee pull up

Session 1075

Ascending Partner amrap 40 min
10 cal bike or row
30 x kB swing

20 cal
30 x kB swing

30 cal
30 x kB swing

40 cal
20 x kB CLEAN & JERK

50 cal
20 x kB clean and jerk

60 cal
20 x kB clean and jerk

70 cal
10 x synchro KB SNATCH

80 cal
10 x synchro snatch

90 cal
10 x synchro snatch

Session 1076

3 rounds for time
10 x burpee over Db's
15 x Db clean and jerk (22.5/15)

Rest

5 rounds for time
5 x hang power clean (70/50)
15 x wallball

Session 1077

Strength/skill:
Front squat 5 x 2
*3 second pause at bottom position

WOD: amrap 8 min
12 x single arm overhead DB lunge (22.5/15)
18 x DB snatch

Rest

1 min max cals assault bike

Session 1078

Strength/skill:
Ring dips 5 x max effort
Or
5 x 10 assisted

WOD: 3 rounds for time
20 x pull up
30 x plate snatch (20/15)
400 m run

Session 1079

Strength/skill:
Hang squat clean - 3/3/2/2/1/1

WOD: 1 min window
25 air squat
Amrap c+j (60/40)
Rest 1 min
Repeat x 8

Session 1080

40 min strongman

Amrap 8 min
10 x renegade row
5 x Db hang squat clean

Session 1081

15/12/9
Cluster (60/40)
L-sit pull up

Rest

Amrap 12
2 x muscle up
4 x jumping lunge (each leg)
8 x kB swing (24/16)

Session 1082

Strength/skill:
Push press - 5 x 5

WOD: amrap 12 min
8 x hspu
16 x wallball
24 x double unders

Session 1083
Strength/skill:
Turkish get up - over 10-12 reps work to a heavy.

WOD: 10-1
TTB
Db box step overs (22,5/15)
*2 x clean and jerk after each round (60/40)

Session 1084

Strength/skill:
Overhead squat - 5 x 3
*3 sec pause at bottom

WOD: 3 min window
15 x pull up
15 x push up
15 x squat

Max effort devils press

Rest 90 sec
Repeat x 5

Session 1086

Strength/skill
Deadlift 5 x 5

WOD: amrap 7 min
6 x Db snatch
2 x burpee box jump
*increase burpee box x each round

Session 1086

Partner Amrap 40 min
5 x synchro med ball clean
5 x synchro push ups

10 x cal bike/row (half each)

10 x synchro ball clean
10 x synchro push ups
20 x cal bike/row (half each)

15 x synchro ball clean
15 x synchro push ups
30 x cal bike/row

20 x synchro ball clean
20 x synchro push ups
40 x cal bike/row

Etc... continue adding 5 reps to cleans and push ups. Cals = combined reps of bike and push ups

Session 1087

5/4/3/2/1
Rope climb
400 m run after each climb

Rest

8 min amrap
12 x Db thruster (22.5/15)
12 x kB sumo high pull (24/16)

Session 1088

Strength/skill:
Weighted pull up - 5 x 5

WOD- for time
100 x double under
4 x clean and jerk (70/45)
50 x sit up
3 x clean and jerk
75 x box jump
2 x clean and jerk
50 x sit up

1 x clean and jerk
100 x double under

Session 1089
Strength/skill:
Back squat 3 x 10

WOD: 3 rounds for time
30 x wallball
20 x ttb
10 x front rack lunge (40/30)

Session 1090

Strength/skill:
Power clean 5 x 3
*reset each rep, light and snappy 70% 'Ish

WOD: Ascending ladder 15 min
Hang power clean x 2 (60/40)
Renegade row x 2
*increase x 2 reps

Session 1091

Strength/skill:
Strict press 4 x 7

WOD: 2 rounds for time
30 x burpee
25 x kB swing (24/16)
20 x thruster (40/30)
15 x pull up

Session 1092

Strength/skill:
3rft
21 x wallball
15 x hspu
9 x ttb

Rest

21/15/9
Hang power snatch (40/30)
Chest to bar pull up

Session 1093
1 - c & j (70/5 0)
2 - thruster
3 - man maker (22.5/15)
4 - Db lunges
5 - wallball
6 - deadlift
7 - burpees
8 - hang power clean
9- deadball over shoulder
10- back squat
11- 1.1k run
12- front squat

Session 1094

Strength/skill:
Ring dips - 5 x max effort

WOD: 2 min window
30 x double unders
10 x burpee
Max single arm Db hang clean and jerk
Rest 1 min repeat
Continue untill 60 Db clean and jerks complete.
*capped at 7 rounds

Session 1095
Strength/skill:
Push press 1rm

WOD: Amrap 7 min
20 x push up
20 x KB sumo high pull (24/16)

Rest 3 min

Amrap - 7 min
10 x pull up
20 x sit up

Session 1096
Strength/skill:
Front squat 1rm

WOD: 3 rounds for time
1a2 x cluster (60/40)
15 x ttb
18 x Db snatch (22.5/15)

Session 1097

40 min strongman

WOD: amrap 10 min
7 x pull up
10 x push
7 x wallball

Session 1098

3 rounds for time
400m run
15 x thruster (40/30)
3 x rope climb

Rest

For time
25 x pull up
25 x burpee
50 x burpee pull up

Session 1099
Strength/skill:
Dynamic effort box squat
10 x 3 @ 65% EMOM

WOD: 18 min ascending ladder
2 x Db box step overs (22.5/15)
2 x Db burpee deadlift
2 x box jump
*increase x 2

Session 1100
Strength/skill:
Bench press 3rm

WOD: for time
75 x sit up
50 x Db snatch (22.5/15)
10 x DB squat clean (AHAP)
50 x Db snatch
75 x sit up

Session 1101

Strength/skill:
Power clean 3rm

WOD: for time
400m run
9 x hang clean and jerk (60/40)
400m run
12 x hang clean and jerk
400m run
15 x hang clean and jerk
400m run

Session 1102

Strength/skill:
Front squat 3rm
Back squat - 20 reps @ 80% - 10kg

WOD: amrap 12
120 x wallball
30 x muscle up
*scaled to burpee pull-ups

Session 1103

40 min AMRAP

100 cal bike/row
100 x single arm thrusters
50 cal bike/row
50 x Db snatch
25 cal bike/row
25 x synchro sit ups

Session 1104

2 rounds for time
80 x double unders
40 x air squat
20 x deadlift (80/60)

Rest

9/15/21
Hang power clean (60/40)
Box jump

Session 1105

Strength/skill:
Dynamic effort box squat
12 x 2 @ 55%

WOD: 3 min window
400m run
Max effort burpee pull up
Rest 1 min
Repeat x 5 rounds

Session 1106
Strength/skill:
Weighted ring dips - 5 x 5

WOD: 10 rounds for time
20 x kb swing (24/16)
15 x sit up
2 x Turkish get up (15/10)

Session 1107

Strength/skill:
Hang power snatch work to heavy 3

WOD: 12 min amrap
1 x power snatch (50/35) *increase x1
10 x push up
25 x double under

Session 1108

Front squat- 5rm
Back squat 20 reps 80% - 15kg

WOD: 3 rounds for time
20 x right arm oh Db lunge (22.5/15)
10 x Ttb
20 x left arm oh Db lunge
10 x pull up

Session 1109
40 min strongman

10 min ascending ladder
2 x air squat
2 x burpee
2 x Db snatch

*increase reps x 2 each round

Session 1110

5 rounds for time
9 x thruster (50/35)
1 x legless rope climb

Rest

7 rounds for time
7 x hspu
6 x pull up
5 x hang power snatch (50/35)

Session 1111
Strength/skill:
Dynamic effort box squat
10 x 2 @ 70% Emom

WOD: for time
50 x box jump
1 x cluster (70/47.5)
50 x push up
2 x cluster
50 x wallball
3 x cluster
50 x KTE
4 x cluster

Session 1112

Strength/skill:
Power clean 5 x 1

WOD: amrap 12 min

8 x Sumo high pull (60/40)
32 x sit ups
100m overhead plate carry (20/15)

Session 1113

Strength/skill:
Push press -work to 2rm
Then 2 extra sets of 2 @ 90%

WOD: every 3 min start a new round x 6 rounds
10 x burpee
12 x double DB hang snatch (22.5/15)
10 x pull up (*incease x 1 each round)

Strength/skill:
Front squat heavy 2
Back squat x 20 reps @ 80% -20kg

WOD: 10 - 1 reps of
DB power clean (22.5/15)
DB lunge (in rack position)
*reps per leg, e.g 10 reps EACH leg

Session 1114

40 min partner amrap
Partner A - 400m run
Partner B - chip away at list
Swap upon partner A return

50 x Man makers
50 x sit ups
50 cal bike / row
50 x devils press

50 x sit ups
50 cal bike / row

Session 1115

Amrap 12
1 x round of Cindy
1 x round of DT

*cindy - 5 x pull up, 10 x push up, 15 x squat
*DT - 12 x deadlift, 9 x hang power clean, 6 x push jerk (70/45)

Rest

For time
100 x burpee
Emom 5 x ttb

Session 1116

Strength/skill:
Dynamic effort box squat
10 x 2 @60%

WOD: 2 min window
2 x bear complex (40/30)
Max effort box jump

Rest 2 min
Repeat x 6 rounds
*increase complex x 1 each round
*if can't complete reps of complex in time frame go back a rep

Session 1117

Strength/skill:
Snatch grip deadlift- 5 x 5

WOD: amrap 10 min
80 x double unders

20 x DB snatch (22.5/15)
10 x burpee over Db

Session 1118

Strength/skill:
Pull up 4 x max effort
Or
Accumulate 15-20 negative reps

WOD: 3 rounds for time
12 x renegade row (22.5/15)
800m run

Strength/skill:
Front squat
heavyish 3rep

Back squat 20 reps. 5kg heavier than last week. (Should be 80% - 25kg)

WOD: for time
200 walking lunges (*can jump)
Emom 1 x cluster (60/40)

Session 1119

40 min strongman

WOD: amrap 10 min
20 x kB swing
20 x sit ups
20 x jumping lunges

Session 1120

9 rounds for time
1 x clean and jerk (75%)
3 x l-sit pull up
5 x ring dips
7 x DB lunge (22.5/15)

Rest

For time
50 x burpee box overs

Session 1121
Strength/skill:
Dynamic effort Box squat (just below parallel) - 10 x 2 @ 50% EMOM

WOD: 90 sec window
3 x sumo high pull (40/30)
3 x thruster
3 x hang power clean
Max effort double unders

90 sec rest
Repeat x 7 rounds
*increase x 1 rep every round
*if you get to a round you can't complete all barbell movements go back a rep

Session 1122

Strength/skill:
Bench press - 5 x 3 (pause on chest each rep)

WOD: amrap 12 min
10 x Db box step over (22.5/15)
15 x box jump
E2mom - 3 x clean and jerk (60/40)

Session 1123

Strength/skill:
Find heavy complex-
Power snatch/overhead squat/hang squat snatch

WOD: 3 rounds for time

24 x Db snatch (22.5/15)
16 x burpee
8 x ttb

Session 1124

Strength/skill:
Front squat - heavyish 5
Back squat 1 x 20 (starting weight is 80% of 1rm then - 30kg)
*(will be adding 5kg each week)

WOD - 20.5

Session 1125

In pairs
40 min clock
200 cal row/bike

Into amrap in remainder
60 x burpee over partner
60 x synchro KB clean & jerk

30 x burpee over partner
30 x plate snatch

100 x synchro devils press

Session 1126

10-1
Pull up strict
Strict press (35/25)
Box jump

Rest

5 rounds for time
15 x power clean (40/30)

15 x wallball

Session 1127
Strength/skill:
Hang power clean 5 x 2

WOD: 12 min amrap
12 x overhead lunge (40/30)
15 x TTB
27 x double unders

Session 1128

Strength/skill:
Strict press 3x3
Push press 3x3

WOD: for time
15 x rounds of "Cindy"

5 x pull
10 x push up
15 x squat

Emom - 6 x Db snatch

Session 1129

40 min strongman

WOD: amrap 10 min
12 x medball clean
12 x push up
12 x ring row

Session 1130

15/12/9/6/3
DB burpee
DB thruster

Rest

21/15/9
DB snatch
Pull up

If time allows
Secret Bonus WOD

Session 1131

Strength/skill:
Clean and jerk - work to 2rm

WOD: amrap 9 min
2 x Hang power clean (60/40)
10 x box jump
*increase clean x2 each round

Session 1132
Strength/skill:
Pendlay row 5 x 5

WOD: for time
75 x wallball
150 x sit up
75 x wallball

Session 1133
Strength/skill:
Overhead lunge - 3 x 10 (5 each leg)

WOD: 8 rounds for time
8 x burpee
100m run
8 x pull up
100m run

Session 1134
Strength/skill:
Push press 5 x 5

WOD : open WOD 20.3
21/15/9
Deadlift (102/70)
Hspu
Into
21/15/9
Deadlift
Handstand walk 50ft

9min cap

Session 1135

5 rounds for time
50 double double
15 x push press (35/25
10 x toes to bar

Rest

For time
50 x Db burpee deadlift (22.5/15)

Session 1136

Strength/skill:
Deficit deadlift 3 x 3 AHAP

WOD: 3 min window
10 x pull up
10 x burpee
10 x kB swing (24/16)
Max effort jumping lunge holding medball

Rest 60 sec
Repeat x 5 rounds

*if you have longer than 30 sec of lunges
Increase reps x 2

Session 1137
Weighted Ring dip 5 x 5

WOD: amrap 20min
30 x sit up
15 x box jump
2 x single arm DB cluster (22.5/15)
*incease cluster x2 each round

Session 1138
Strength/skill:
Squat snatch - work up to heavy

WOD: 3 rounds for time
10 x hang clean and jerk (50/35)
800m run

Session 1139
3 rounds for time
20 x thruster (40/30)
15 x ttb
10 x hang power clean

Rest

Amrap 14 min
50 x double under
12 x sumo high pull (40/30)
2 x rope climb

Session 1140
Strength/skill:
Overhead squat 5 x 3

WOD: for time
50 x devils press (22.5/15)
Emom - 5 x box jump

Session 1141

Strength/skill:
Pendlay row - 5x5

WOD: 5 rounds for time
12 x pull up
18 x wallball

Session 1142

Strength/skill:
Db push jerk 5 x 5 (single arm)

WOD: amrap 20 min
12 x hspu
24 x kB swing (24/16)
36 x o/h kB lunge

Session 1143

For time as a 2 person team

400 x double unders
200 x sit ups
100 x squat clean
50 x rope climb

Session 1144

Strength/skill:
Push jerk 5 x 3

WOD: amrap 12 min
Deadlift x 5 (100/70)
Kb clean and jerk x 10 (24/16)
Push up x 15

Session 1145

Strength/skill:
Front rack lunge- 4 x 10m

WOD: 5 rounds for time
20 x wallball
10 x box jump
20 x sit up

Session 1146
Strength/skill:
1rm bench press

WOD: 10 rounds for time
5 x Db hang power clean (22.5/15)
5 x burpee over Db
5 x pull up

Session 1147
Strength/skill:
Hang squat clean - 2rm

WOD: amrap 14 min

Clean and jerk x 1
Toes to bar x 10
Double under x 50

*increase clean and jerk x 1

Session 1149

4 rounds for time
25 x thruster (20/15)
5 x ring muscle up

Rest

4 rounds for time

24 x front rack lunge (30/25)
18 x hang power clean
12 x push jerk

Session 1149

Strength/skill:
Sumo high pull - 5 x 5

WOD: amrap - 9 min
1 x Hang power snatch (40/30)
5 x bar over burpee
*increase snatch x 1 each round

Session 1150
Strength/skill:
Weighted pull up 5 x 5

WOD: 30/20/10
Renegade row (22.5/15) *no push up
Plate snatch (20/15)
100m over head plate carry after each round

Session 1151

Strength/skill:
1 rm strict press

WOD: amrap 5 min
3 x power clean (60/40)
6 x push up
9 x air squat
Rest 1 min
Repeat x 4 rounds

Session 1152
Strength/skill:
Squat clean 3rm

WOD:

WOD: for time
50 x ttb
5 x dball squat clean (ahap)
50 x kB swing
4 x dball squat clean
50 x sit ups
3 x dball squat clean
50 x hollow rocks
2 x dball squat clean
50 x v -ups
1 x dball squat clean

Session 1153

Strength/skill:
Deadlift 1rm

WOD: 2 min window
12 x HR push up
12 x DB Snatch (22.5/15)
Max effort wallball

1 min rest
Repeat x 5 rounds

Session 1154

Strength/skill:
L - sit: accumulate 3 min
Ring dip support: accumulate 3 min

WOD: amrap 25 min
400m run
12 x Turkish ups (15/10)
24 x single Db hang clean and jerk (same Db, alternating)

Session 1155

Strength/skill:
Hang power snatch 2rm

WOD: 5 rounds for time
15 x kb swing (24/16)
10 x pull up
5 x ttb
50 x double unders

Session 1156

Strength/skill:
Ring dip 12/10/8/6 (add weight accordingly)

Or 5 x 10 banded

WOD: for time
3 rounds for time
15 x sumo high pull (40/30)
20 x toes bar
25 x deadball over shoulder
800m run

Session 1157

Strength/ skill:
Strict press 3x5 @70%

WOD: 3 rounds for time
Buy in/out 100 x double unders
12 x devils press (22.5/15)
24 x pull up

Session 1158

Strength squat Deload

WOD: amrap 15 min
8 x power clean (60/40)
12 x front rack lunge

16 x box jump

Session 1159

3 rounds for time
50 x double unders
20 x wallball
15 x power snatch (35/25)

Rest

4 rounds for time
14 x hspu
7 x squat clean (80/55)

Session 1160

Strength/ skill:
Deadlifts 10 x 1 @65% plus bands EMOM

WOD: 3 min window
30 x air squat
30 x Db hang power clean (22.5/15)
Max effort burpee pull up
Rest 2 min
Repeat x 4

Session 1161
Strength/skill::
Pull up negatives accumulate 15 - 20 reps

WOD: for time

10 x man maker (22.5/15)
40 x sit up
5 x man maker
40 x sit ups
10 x man maker

Session 1162

Strength/skill:
Bench press 10 x 3 @70% (speed focus)

WOD: 21/18/15/12
Bar facing burpee
Push press (40/30)

Session 1163

Strength- squat

WOD AMRAP 10 min
5 x B.B. complex squat clean/ lunge (50/35)
10 x box jump

Session 1164
Strongman

WOD: 10 min amrap
24 x double under
12 x Db power snatch
6 x burpee pull up

Session 1165

Running Jackie
1000m run
50 x thruster (20/15)
30 x pull up

Rest

4 rounds for time
100m farmer carry (22.5/15)
14 x hspu
10 x Db squat

Session 1166

Strength/skill:
Overhead squat 3 x 5

WOD: 5 rounds each for time
6 x deadlift @70%
6 x box jumps
6 x burpees
6 x burpee box jump

Rest 1 min

Session 1167

Strength/skill:
Ring row 5 x 10 (elevated feet of possible)

WOD: for time
20 x renegade rows (22.5/15)
40 x ttb

15 x renegade row
20 x ttb

10 x renegade row
10 x ttb

Session 1168
Strength/skill:
Strict press 2RM
Then 3 x 2 @90% of above

WOD: 3 rounds for time
15 x hang clean and jerk (40/30)
10 x sumo high pull
400m run

Session 1169

Strength squatting hypertrophy

WOD.: amrap 10 min
30 x oh Db lunge
30 x kB swing

Session 1170

Partner amrap 30 min
20 x thruster (50/35)
20 x burpee box jump

30 x thruster (40/30)
30 x burpee box jump

40 x thruster (30/20)
40 x burpee box jump

50 x thruster (20/15)
50 x burpee box jump

Max distance bike/row in remainder time

*1 partner working at a time (swap as needed)

Session 1171

50 x double unders
50 x back squat (40/30)
50 x toes to bar
50 x double unders
50 x bar facing burpee
50 x push press
50 x double unders
50 x wallball
50 x pull-up
50 x double unders
50 x push up
50 x sit up
50 x double unders

Session 1172

Strength/skill:
Deadlift 2rm

WOD: 1 min window
5 x sumo high pull (60/40)
10 x push up
Max box jumps in remainder
Rest 30 sec
Repeat x 10 rounds

Session 1173

Strength/skill:
Db power snatch 5 x 3 each arm

WOD: for time
75 x lunge
75 x sit ups
9 x Turkish get up (15/10)

50 x lunge
50 x sit up
6 x Turkish get up

25 x lunge
25 x sit up
3 x Turkish get up

Session 1174

Strength/skill:
Bench press - 12/10/8/8

WOD: 5 rounds for time
12 x pull up
6 x clean and jerk (60/40)
400m run

Session 1175
Squats -speed

WOD amrap 10 min
8 x Db box step overs
8 x Db thruster

Session 1176

Strongman

WOD: 10 min amrap
8 x single Db clean and jerk
20 x sit ups

Session 1177

Death by thruster (40/30)

Rest

12/9/6
L-sit pul up
Hspu
Burpee
Deadball over shoulder

Session 1178

Strength/skill:
Deadlift deload: 3 x 5 @ 65-70%

WOD: 90 sec window
30 x double under
12 x o/h plate lunge
Max Db hang squat clean
Rest 30 sec

Repeat x 7 rounds

Session 1179

Strength/skill:
Strict press 3 x 5 @65-70%

WOD: amrap 20 min
12 x DB snatch (22.5/15)
9 x box jump
6 x ttb

Session 1180
Strength/skill:
Power clean - 5/5/3/3/1/1
*touch and go reps

WOD:
10-1 Burpees
2 x clean and jerk after each round (70/50)

Session 1181

Strength
Squat

WOD: for time

40 x wallball
15 x pull up

30 x wallball
15 x pull up

20 x wallball
15 x pull ups

Session 1182

30 min partner amrap
100 x O/h Db lunges
100 x Db snatch
100 x single Db clusters

Partner A chips away at reps
Partner B rows or bikes 12/8 cals then swap

Rest

7 min amrap
1 for 1 burpee pull up

Session 1183

15/12/9
Clean and jerk (60/40)
Pull up

Rest

"Db Elizabeth "
21/15/9
Squat clean (22.5/15)
Ring dip

Session 1184

Deadlift 8 x 2 @ 60% with band
*1 min rest

WOD: 1 min window
10 x burpees over Db
Max Db snatch in remainder (22.5/15)
Rest 30 sec

Repeat x 10 rounds

Session 1185

Strength/skill:
Emom 10 min
5-8 strict pull ups

WOD: for time
70 x sit ups
60 x Kb swing (24/16)
10 x squat clean (80/55)
50 x KB swing
40 x sit up

Session 1186
Strength/skill:
Bench press 2 x 8
1 x max

WOD: for time
Hang power snatch x 25 (40/30)
Double under x 50

Hang power snatch x 15 (50/35)
Double under x 100

Hang power snatch x 5 (60/40)
Double double x 150

Session 1187

Strength
Squats

WOD: Ascending ladder 7 min
db burpee box step ups
8 x lunges

Add 1 rep to step ups

Session 1188

40 min strongman

WOD: partner amrap 10 min
30 x synchro medball cleans
30 x partner clap push up

Session 1189

Amrap 7 min
20 x double unders
7 x Db power clean (22.5/15)

Rest 3 min

Amrap 7 min
10 x ring dip
7 x deadball ground to overhead

Rest 3 min

Amrap 7 min
20 x kB swing (24/16)
7 x burpee pull up

Session 1190

Strength/skill:
Deadlift 5rm

WOD: 90 second window
14 x front rack lunge (40/30)
Max effort wallballs
Rest 30 seconds repeat x 6 rounds

Session 1191

Strength/skill:
Pull up negatives - 20 reps
Add weight or band to achieve a 3-5 second negative.

WOD: 10-1
Burpee box jump
Turkish get up (15/10)

Session 1192

Strength/skill
Strict press 9 x 3 @60% (speed focus)

WOD: 7 rounds for time
8 x hspu
9 x hang power clean (60/40)
10 x TTB

Session 1193

Strength/skill:
Squat hypertrophy

WOD: amrap 8 min

18x Single Db cluster (22.5/15)
12x push up

Session 1194

For time
9 x thruster (40/30)
9 x box jump
400m run
12 x thruster
12 x box jump
400m run
15 x thruster
15 x box jump

400m run
18 x thruster
18 x box jump
400m run
21 x thruster
21 x box jump
400m run

Session 1195

Strength/skill:
Accumulate 3 min in L-sit
Accumulate 3 min in ring support

WOD: 4 min window
20 x pull up
20 x Kb sumo high pull (24/16)
Max effort devil press (22.5/15)

Rest 90 sec repeat x 4 rounds

Session 1196

Strength/skill:
Bench press 5rm

WOD: 27/21/15/9
Bar facing burpee
Overhead lunges (40/30)

Session 1197
Strength/skill:
Power clean 3rm
Then 5 min emom- 1 Rep @ 3rm weight

WOD: for time

15 x hang clean and jerk (60/40)

25 x ttb
35 x box jump
25 x ttb
15 x hang clean and jerk

Session 1198

Strongman 40 min

WOD: 10 min amrap
10 x renegade row
20 x air squat

Session 1199

18/15/12/9/6/3
Single Db box step overs (22.5/15)
Db snatch

Rest

4 rounds for time
15 x pull up
5 x hang squat clean (80/55)

Session 1200
Strength/skill:
Sumo Deadlift 3 x 5 @ 70%

WOD: 3 min window
20 x wallball
10 x ttb
20 x double unders
Max sit ups

Rest 1 min repeat x 5 rounds

Session 1201
Strength/skill:
Weighted dips 8/6/4/6/8
Dball chest pass x 3 to wall after each set

WOD: for time
Hspu x 30
Dball ground to overhead x 30
Db hang snatch x 30 (22.5/15) *2 dbs
Dball ground to overhead x30
Hspu x 30

Session 1202
Strength/skill:
Push press 10 x 3 @65%
*1 min rest, aim to move bar fast!

WOD: ascending ladder 7 min
3 x sumo high pull (50/35)
3 x burpee pull up
Increase x 3

Rest 2 min

Repeat
*start reps from where you finished first amrap

Session 1203
Strength
Back squat deload

WOD: 3 rounds for time
18 x thruster (40/30)
18 x box jump
18 x kB swing

Session 1204

20 min amrap
In teams
100 cal bike or row
100 Db box step ups

100 push-ups
100 over head Db lunge

Rest 10 min

Amrap 20 min
In teams
100 cal bike or row
100 ring row
100 sit ups
100 burpees

Session 1205

3 rounds for time
21 x wallball
15 x pull ups
9 x power snatch (40/30)

Rest

12 min ascending ladder
Turkish get up (15/10)
10 x single Db hang clean and jerk
*increase reps by 1

Session 1206

Strength/skill:
Overhead squat - 5rm

WOD: 10 rounds for time

3 x deadlift (140/100)
5 x squat with Db in left rack (22.5/15)
5 x squat with Db in right rack

Session 1207
Strength/skill:

Weighted pull up 8/6/4/6/8
Or
Accumulate 20 negative reps for quality

WOD: amrap 20 min
40 x renegade rows (15/10) *no push up
40 x kB sumo high pull (24/16)
30 x left arm Db push press
30 x right arm Db push press
20 x ttb
20 x sit up

Session 1208

Strength/skill:
Bench press 4 x 8

WOD: 3 rounds for time
40 x double unders
20 x burpee
10 x clean and jerk (50/35)

Session 1209

Strength
Box squat
Front squat

WOD: amrap 8 min
20 x Db box step over
20 x wallball

Session 1210

40 min strongman

WOD: 10 min partner amrap
30 x synchro med ball clean
30 x partner medball sit up

Session 1211
3 rounds for time
20 x thruster (35/25)
2 x rope climb

Rest

For time
15/12/9/6 reps
DB snatch (22.5/15)
Burpee over Db
Hspu
Knees to elbow

Session 1212
Deadlift - 8 x 2 @ 50% (+ bands)
*speed focus, move bar fast. 1 min rest

WOD: 4 min window
10 x Db deadlift (22.5.15)
20 x Db hang power clean
30 x sit up
Max single arm overhead Db lunge
Rest 2 min
Repeat x 4 rounds

Session 1213
Strength/skill:
Db snatch 5 x 2 each arm

WOD: amrap 20 min
30 x Squat clean (60/40)
30 x burpee to 6" target

Session 1214
Strength/skill:
Strict press 5 x 3

WOD: for time
100 x double unders
80 x plate snatch (20/15)
60 x push up
40 x Db S2O (22.5/15)
20 x C2B
100 x double unders

Session 1214

Strength/skill:
Box squat 2 x 10@ 72%
1 x max @ 72%

Front squat 4 x 8 @ 70%

WOD: amrap 10 min
Front rack lunge x 12 (40/30)
TTB x 12
Hang power clean x 12

Session 1215

Partner WOD

Amrap 10 min
8 x Db thruster (15/10)
8 x ring row

Rest 2 min

Amrap 10 min
8 x Db snatch
8 x box jump

Rest 2 min

Amrap 10 min
8 x Db clean and jerk

8 x push up

*each workout follows a "you go I go" format

Session 1216

21/15/9
Power clean (40/30)
Overhead squat

Rest

5 rounds for time
15 x Kb swing (24/16)
15 x burpee

Session 1217
Strength/skill:
Hang power clean 5 x 2

WOD: amrap 8 min
50 x sit up
8 x bar muscle up

Rest 2 min

Amrap 6 min
4 x renegade row (22.5/15)
8 x TTB

Session 1218
Strength/skill:
Deadlift - 3rm

WOD: 2 min window
20 x Db front rack lunges (22.5/15)
Max effort box jumps
Rest 1 min repeat x 5 rounds

Session 1219
Strength/skill:
Ring dips - 5 x 10
Superset
Ring row

WOD: 50/40/30/20/10
Push press (40/30)
Double unders (reps x2)

Session 1220

Strength/skill:
Back squat 6 x 3 @ 62.5% (1 min rest, think about moving fast! Dynamic effort)

Front squat Emom x 10 @ 70% (

WOD: amrap 10 min
2 x devil press (15/10)
7x pull up
7 x wallball

4 x devil press
7 x pull up
7 x wallball

Session 1221
30 min clock
120 x burpee
Then in remainder time
Ascending ladder x 2's
2 x strict pull ups
2 x clusters (40/30)

4x strict pull ups
4 x clusters

Etc.......

Session 1222

Strength/skill:
Weighted pull ups work to 5rm then 2 x max sets unweighted
*if you don't have pull ups accumulate 15 negatives then 2 banded sets for max reps

WOD: 4 min window
30 x wallball
8 x hang power clean (60/40)
Max Db burpee deadlift box step ups
Rest 2 min repeat x 4 rounds

*cleans in no more than 2 sets

Session 1223
Strength/skill:
Push press waves - 5/3/5/3/5/3

WOD: for time
75 x sit up
40 x hspu
75 x sit up

Session 1224
Strength/skill:
Front squat waves - 5/3/5/3/5/3

WOD: amrap 8 min
12 x Pull up
6 x DB cluster (22.5/15)

Session 1225
Strength/skill:
Bench press 3 x 5
Superset
Pendlay row 3 x 5

WOD: for time
20 x burpee
4 x bear complex (50/35)
20 x burpee

3 x bear complex
20 x burpee
2 x bear complex
20 x burpee
1 x bear complex

Session 1226

5 rounds for time
50 x double unders
5 x squat clean (70/50)

Rest

9/15/21
Push jerk (50/35)
Hspu
Ttb

Session 1227
Strength/skill:
Overhead squat- 5 x 3

WOD: 3 min window
30 x single arm O/H Db lunge (22.5/15)
Max renegade rows
Rest 2 min repeat x 4 rounds

Session 1228
Strength/skill:
Strict press - 5 x 5

WOD: 12 min clock
3 min of Db snatch
3 min of burpee pull ups
2 min of Db snatch
2 min of burpee pull ups
1 min of Db snatch
1 min of burpee pull ups

Session 1229
Strength/skill:
hang power snatch heavy 2

WOD: amrap 12 min
40 x Kb swing 24/16)
30 x Clean and jerk (40/30)
20 x box jump

Session 1230
Strength/skill:
Sumo high pull- 5 x 3

WOD: for time
60 x double unders
20 x wallball
15 x deadlift (80/55)

90 x double unders
20 x wallball
15 x deadlift

120 x double unders
20 x wallball
15 x deadlift

Session 1231

2 rounds for time
22 x deadlift (100/70)
22 x hspu

Rest

2 rounds for time
22 x ttb
22 x hang power snatch

Session 1232

Strength/skill:
Power clean - find heavy 3

WOD - amrap 20 min
Box jump x 20
Power clean x 15 (60/40)

Session 1233
Strength/skill:
Bench press- 8/6/4/8/6/4

WOD: for time
75 x double unders
30 x Turkish get up (15/10)
75 x double under

Session 1234

Strength/skill:
Front squat- 8/8/6/6

WOD: "Fran"
21/15/9
Thruster (42.5/30)
Pull ups

Session 1235

40 min strongman

WOD: 10 min partner amrap
3 x Db hang clean and jerk
3 x Db burpee deadlift

*you go I go

Session 1236

2 rounds for time
50 x front rack lunge (40/30)
4 x rope climb

Rest

Amrap 15 min
15 x pull ups
15 x clean and jerk (40/30)
15 x kB swing (24/16)

Session 1237
Strength/skill:
Db snatch 4 x 3 each arm

WOD: 5 min window
20 x hang squat clean (50/35)
20 x ttb
20 x burpee
Max Db box step ups
2 min rest
Repeat x 5 rounds
*if you fail to get to step ups reduce all reps by 5.

Session 1238

Strength/skill:
3" Deficit deadlift- 4 x 3

WOD:
4/3/2/1/2/3/4
Man makers (22,5/15) (no push up)
8 x box jump after each round

Session 1239
Strength/skill:
hang power snatch + power snatch. Work to heavy

WOD: 2 rounds for time

4 x power clean (70/50)
5 x front squat
6 x push jerk
40 x pull ups
50 x sit ups
60 x push ups

Session 1240

Strength/skill:
Thruster- work to heavy single then 5rm then 7rm

WOD: amrap 14 min
30 x sumo high pull (40/30)
30 x wallball
100 x double unders

Session 1241

Partner WOD
10 min amrap
10 x DB alternating Db snatch
10 x single arm overhead lunges (5 each arm)

Rest 3 min

Amrap 10 min
40 x wallball
20 x slam ball burpee

Rest 3 min

Amrap 10 min
Max cals bike or row

*for all wods one person works for a minute at a time. Swapping every minute.

Session 1242

2 rounds for time
50m OH plate walk
25 x burpee

Rest 5 min

2 rounds for time
25 x thruster (40/30)
25 x bar facing burpees

Rest 5 min

2 rounds for time
25 x pull up
25 x burpee to target

Session 1243
Strength/skill:
Hang power clean 3/3/2/2/1/1

WOD: EMOM 20 min
3 x power clean (60/40)
3 x front squat
3 x push jerk

If you miss a round amrap untill end

(Rx+ 70/50)

Session 1244

Strength/skill:
1rm weighted dip
Then
3 x max effort sets unweighted

Or

5 sets using bands (use a band that allows 5-7 reps)

WOD: 10 rounds for time
10 x deadlift (60/40)
12 x push up
10 x sit up

Session 1245

Strength/skill:
Back squat 1&1/4's - 4 x 6

WOD: amrap 8 min
8 x burpee box jump
12 x back squat (50/35)
*no rack for squat

Rest 2 min

For time
50 x KB swing (24/16)
10 x thruster (50/35)
25 x Kb swing

Session 1246
Strength/skill:
Strict press work to heavy 3
Push press - 2 x max effort at above weight

WOD:
3 rounds for time
25 x pull up
25 x Db hang power clean
50 x double unders

Session 1247

40 min strongman

WOD: 10 min partner amrap

20 x pull up (partner must hang from bar)
40 x push up (partner must plank)

Session 1248

As pairs get as far you can in 40 min
100 x O/H plate lunge (20/15)
Choose 1 - 1km run/ 1.2km row or 65/45cal bike
80x O/H lunge
Run/row/bike
60 x O/H lunge
Run/row/bike
40 x O/H lunge
Run/row/bike
20 x O/H lunge
Run/row/bike

*divide as needed

Session 1249
Strength/skill:
2 position snatch (hang squat + full snatch). Work to heavy

WOD: 3 min window
35 x wallball
Max effort Turkish get ups (15/10)

Rest 1 min

3 min window
35 x wallball
Max effort Db burpee deadlift (22.5/15)

Rest 2 min repeat

Session 1250

Strength/skill:
Build to heavy single pull up

then 5 x 3 weighted negatives @same weight.

Or if you don't have pull ups yet
Accumulate 20 nice slow negative reps (use bands if need be to achieve a slower rep)

WOD:
10 x sumo high pull (60/40)
30 x ring row
50 x box jump over
70 x sit ups
50 x box jump overs
30 x ring row
10 x sumo high pull

Session 1251

Strength/skill:
Paused Front squat - 7 x 1

WOD: amrap 12 min
18 x alternating single arm Db cluster (22.5/15)
10 x TTB

Session 1252

Strength/skill:
Bench press 3x5
S/s
Bent over row

WOD:
1/2/3/4/5/4/3/2/1
Muscle up
Clean and jerk (70/50)

Session 1253
40 min partner amrap

75 x pull up
75 x front rack lunges (40/30)
6 x 200m sprints
75 x back squat
75 x push up

*1 partner working at a time. Swap every minute

Session 1254

Amrap 10 min
6 x pull-up
5 x burpee
4 x hang power clean (50/35)
3 x thruster

Rest

4 rounds for time
400m run
7 x hang squat snatch (40/30)
3 x rope climb

Session 1255
Strength/skill:
Deadlift - 3 x 5

WOD: 3 rounds for time
3 x SQUAT clean (85/57.5)
15 x Db push jerk left arm (22.5/15)
3 x POWER clean
15 x Db push jerk right arm

Session 1256
Strength/skill:
3 min Hanging L-sit in as little sets as possible

3 min ring support (push down hard into rings, don't let shoulders shrug. Use bands if need be)

WOD: 10-1
Renegade row (no push up)
Pull up
Db hang power clean

Session 1257
Strength/skill:
Back squat 3 x 5 (3.2.x.1)
*nothing to heavy today just greasing the groove for upcoming squat cycle.

*2 x depth jumps after each set.

WOD: for time
50 x sit up
75 x KB swing (24/16)
100 x bodyweight walking lunge
150 x double unders
100 x walking lunges
75 x Kb swing
50 x sit ups

Session 1258

Strength/skill:
Clean and jerk heavy single
Amrap 5 min triples at 70%

WOD: in a 5 min window complete
7 rounds of:
6 x Db snatch
6 x push up
6 x box jump
Then max burpee in remainder

Rest 2 min repeat

Session 1259

40 min strongman

WOD: 10 min partner WOD
1 partner working for a minute at a time

14 x O/h plate lunge (20/15)
Max single arm alternating Db cluster

Session 1260

5 rounds for time
9 x bar facing burpees
6 x hspu
3 x deadlift @ 75%

Rest

3 rounds for time
15 x pull ups
15 x hang power snatch (40/30)

Session 1261
Strength/skill:
Bench press - work to heavy triple
3 x max effort sets @ 80% of above

WOD: for time
30 x man makers (22.5/15)

Session 1262
Strength/skill:
Front rack walking lunges 4 x 12 steps

WOD: for time
100 x Db box step overs (22.5/15)
Emom - 5 x TTB

Session 1263

Strength/skill:
Push jerk - 5/3/3/2/2/1

WOD: amrap 8 min
12 x hang clean strict press (40/30)
12 x sumo high pull

Rest

2 min max effort bike or row

Session 1264
Strength/skill:
Overhead squat 5 x 3

WOD:
5 x 3 min rounds
25 x wallball
25 x double under
Max effort burpee pull ups
Rest 1 min

Session 1265

21/15/9 reps for time
Hspu
Pull up
Med ball clean

Rest

4 rounds for time
15 x wallball
12 x hang power clean (60/40)
9 x box step overs with DB (22.5/15)

Session 1266

Strength/skill:
Ring dips 5 x 5 (add weight to achieve reps or perform negative reps)

*After each set perform 3 x dball chest passes to wall for speed.

WOD: 20 min clock
100 x sit ups
Then amrap in remainder time
50 x double under
20 x alternating DB hang Snatch (22.5/15)
10 x bar muscle up

Session 1267

Strength/skill:
Back rack lunges 4 x 6 each leg (aim to go as heavy as safely possible. May rest
45 sec between legs)

WOD: for time
40 x thruster (30/20)
15 x bar facing burpees
30 x thruster (35/25)
15 x bar facing burpees
20 x thruster (40/30)
15 x bar facing burpees
10 x thruster (50/35)

Session 1268

Strength/skill:
Pull up - 3 x 5 (add weight to achieve rep or perform negatives)

Emom - 8 min
Min 1 - 6/7 strict pull up/ring row
Min 2 - 10 push up

WOD: 8 rounds for time
2 x plate snatch (20/15)
2 x box jump

*increase by 2 reps each round
*perform 1 Turkish get up after each round

Session 1269
Strength/skill:
Squat clean - heavy 2
Amrap 5 min - 3 TnG @90%

WOD: 5 rounds for time
8 x devils press (22.5/15)
12 x ttb

Session 1270
40 min strongman

WOD - partner amrap 10 min
10 x Kb swing (24/15)
5 x burpee
*you go I go format

26/4/19

4 rounds for time
20 x Db farmer lunge (22.5/15)
20 sec l-sit
10 x hspu

rest

3 rounds for time
400m run
15 x deadlift (60/40)
12 x TTB

Session 1271
Strength/skill:
Front squat 1 &1/4's - 5 x 5

WOD: for time

40 x DB front squat (22.5/15)
30 x Db push jerk left arm
30 x Db push jerk right arm
40 x Db front squat
Emom - 20 x double unders

Session 1272
Strength/skill:
Bench press 4 x 3

DB bench press 3 x 8

WOD: for time
15 x burpee pull up
30 x clean and jerk (60/40)
15 x burpee pull up

Session 1273
Strength/skill:
Back rack lunge 6 x 4 each leg
Super set
Pendlay row - 6 x 4

WOD: 5 rounds for time
8 x sumo high pull (60/40)
3 x rope climb
8 x Ttb

Session 1274
Strength/skill:
Overhead complex - 3 x push press/2x push jerk/ 1 x split jerk
5 working sets

WOD: 3 min window
24 x Db snatch (22.5/15)
12 x pull up
Max wall balls in remainder
Rest 2 min repeat x 4 rounds

Session 1275
Strength/skill:
Power clean - work to heavy 2 (can reset reps)

5 min Amrap - 3 touch and go power cleans @ 80% of above

WOD: amrap 12 min
40 x double unders
8 x clean and jerk (50/35)
6 x bar facing burpee

Session 1276

Strength
Front squat 5 x 2 (3.3.x.0)

WOD: 3 rounds for time
30 x box jump
30 x DB lunges

Session 1277
"Helen"
3 rounds for time
400m run
21 x kB swing
12 x pull up

Rest

"Elizabeth"
21/15/9
Squat clean (60/40)
Ring dip

Session 1278
Strength/skill:
Overhead squat- 5x5 (snatch balance first rep if possible)

WOD: amrap 5 min
2 x deadlift (130/90)
6 x lateral bar hops

12 x KTE

Rest 3 min

1 x deadlift (150/105)
6 x later bar hops
12 x TTB

Session 1279

Strength/skill:
Single DB strict press 5x5 each arm

WOD: for time
30 x burpee box jump
30 x push press (40/30)
20 x burpee box jump
20 x push press
Emom- 3 x sumo high pull

Session 1280
Strength/skill:
Back rack lunge 5 x 6 each leg
After sets 1,3,5 perform 3 depth jumps

WOD: 18/12/6/12/18 reps for time
Hang power snatch (40/30)
Wall ball

Session 1281
Strength/skill:
Find heavy cluster in 15 min then rest 2 min and pick a weight you think you
can do 5 touch and go

WOD: amrap 13 min
15 x single Db thruster left arm
20 x HR push up
15 x right arm thruster
20 x pull up

Session 1282
40 min amrap

In pairs or teams

100 cal bike or row (swapping every 30 sec)
100 x burpee box step up (1 rep each at a time)
100 synchro sit ups

Session 1283

12/10/8/6/4
Power clean (50/35)
Thruster
C2b

Rest

2 rounds
800m run
20 x hspu

Session 1284
Strength/skill:
Weighted ring dips -5/5/3/3/1/1

WOD- 3 min window
15 x plate snatch (20/15)
15 x TTB
Max effort renegade rows (no push up)
1 min rest
Repeat x 5 rounds

Session 1285
Strength/skill:
DB snatch- 7 x 3 each arm (aim to go heavy as your form allows)

WOD: 2 rounds for time
22 x box jump
11 x hang power clean 60/40
7 min cap

2 min rest

Death by lunges
Emom
1 lunge each leg
2 lunges each leg
3 lunges each leg
Continue till failure

Session 1286
Strength/skill:
Weighted pull ups 5/5/3/3/1/1

WOD: amrap 18 min
5 x Kb sumo high pull (24/16)
5 x Kb thruster left arm
5 x Kb thruster right arm

2 rounds of Cindy

10 of each Kb movements

2 rounds of Cindy

15 of each kB movements
Etc......

Session 1287

Strength/skill:
Find heavy complex
Power clean/hang squat clean/front squat/ push press/ push jerk

WOD: 3 rounds for time
10 x DB clean and jerk (22.5/15)

25 x wallball

Session 1288

40 min strongman

WOD: 10 min partner amrap
50 x pull up
40 x synchro plate snatch
50 x med ball clean
40 x synchro plate snatch
50 x plate thruster
40 x synchro plate snatch

*divide pull-ups, cleans and thrusters as needed.

Session 1289

5 rounds
4 x squat clean (80/55)
3 x push jerk
2 x rope climb

Rest

3 rounds
20 x power snatch
10 x bar facing burpees

Session 1290

Strength/skill:
Overhead squat- 5 x 5

WOD: for time
70 x double unders
50 x squat
30 x ttb
10 x push press (60/40)
5 x cluster

10 x push press
30 x ttb
50 x squat
70 x double unders

Session 1291

Strength/skill:
5 x 8-10 ring rows (feet elevated if possible)

WOD: 5min
16x Single Db hang clean and jerk
16x Db box step overs
16x Db lunges (8 each leg)
Max effort burpee box jump

Rest 1 min
Repeat x 4 rounds

Session 1292

Strength/skill:
Hang power clean 5/5/4/4/3/3/2/1

WOD: amrap 12 min
Deadlift x 5 (100/70)
HR push up x 10
Sit up x 15

25/3/19Session 1293
Strength/skill:
Push ups on rings 5 x 8-10

Session 1294

40 min partner amrap

200 cal bike/row
300 wallballs
200 hang power snatch (30/20)

100 bar facing burpee

Session 1295

Strength/skill:
Deadlift 1RM

WOD: 10 - 1
Lunges (each leg)
TTB
medball cleans

Session 1296
Strength/skill:
Bench press 1RM

WOD: amrap 15 min

10 x Renegade row (22.5/15)
12 x single DB clean & jerk (alternating)
50 x double under

Session 1297

Strength/skill:
Front squat 1RM

WOD: 21/15/9
Thruster (50/35)
Box jump

Session 1298

40 min strongman

WOD: partner amrap 10 min

20 x partner clap push up
20 x partner sit up with med ball
20 x partner wallball

Session 1299

4 rounds for time
3 x squat clean (90/60)
15 x kB swing (24/16)
10 x bar facing burpees

Rest

Amrap 12 min
1 round of "DT"
400m run

Session 1300

Strength/skill:
Strict press 3RM

3 rounds not for time
10 x pendlay row
10 x Db strict press

WOD: amrap 3 min
6 x sumo high pull (40/30)
6 x push press
30 x double unders
Rest 1 min
Repeat x 4 rounds

Session 1301
Strength/skill:

Front squat 3RM
back squat 1 x max effort @ 90% of above

WOD: for time

40 x wallball
Into
2 rounds
15 x hang clean and jerk (60/40)
15 x bar over burpee
Into
40 x wallball

Session 1302

*repeat

Team WOD:
In teams of 3 or 4

Amrap 40 min
300 cal bike/row (swapping every 30 sec)
400 m walk with - deadball and 3 kbs
(Deadball can carry however you like, person with 2 kbs must farmer carry,
person with 1 kb must rack carry. Swap as needed)

Session 1303

27/21/15/9
Wallball
Pull ups

Rest

3 rounds for time
14 x hspu
7 x sumo high pull (60/40)

Session 1304

Strength/skill:
Deadlift - 5rm

WOD: amrap 8 min

12 x burpee box jump
12 x Db hang power clean (22.5/15)

Session 1305
Strength/skill:
Push jerk - 5x3

WOD: 30 min to get as close to 1

15 x Db push jerk left arm (22.5/15)
15 x Db push jerk right arm
15 x KB swing (24/16)
15 x sit up

(Then 14 of each, then 13 of each, 12, 11 etc..)

Session 1306
Strength/skill:
Front squat 5RM
Then
1 max effort set back squat @90% of 5rm weight

WOD: 20 min emom
Minute 1- 1 round of Cindy
Minute 2- 2 x power clean and jerk

Session 1307

Strength/spresskill:
Bench press 5rm

WOD:
5 rounds for time
25 x ttb
50 x double unders
15/13/11/9/7 squat clean

Session 1308

6 rounds for time
3 x power snatch (50/35)
2 rounds of Cindy
1 x rope climb

Rest

5 rounds for time
15 x GHD sit ups or 20 sit ups
5 x muscle ups or 10 burpee pull ups

Session 1309
Strength/skill:
Deadlift 7 x 3 @ 60% (speed focus)

WOD: amrap 20 min
6 x devils press (22.5/15)
8 x Db thruster
10 x TTB
12 x walking lunges

Session 1310

Strength/skill:
Push press 7 x 3 (speed focus 90% of STRICT press)

WOD: 10 rounds for time
5 x renegade rows (22.5/15)
7 x pull-up

Session 1311

Strength/skill:
Hang power 5 x 3

WOD: for time
75 x kB swing (24/16)

50 x box jump
25 x hang power clean (70/45)
50 x box jump
75 x kB swing

Session 1312

Strength/skill:
Seated box jump x 20

Front squat 3 x 3 @ 75%

Back squat 2 x 8 @ 60%

WOD : 19.1

Session 1313

40 min strongman

WOD: 10 min partner amrap
50 x Db thruster
200m wallball run/jog
50 x burpee box strep up
200m wallball run/jog

Session 1314

3 rounds for time
15 x front squat (70/45)
12 x TTB
9 x hspu

Rest

4 rounds for time
400m run
15 x KB swing (24/16)
20 x sit up

Session 1315
Strength/skill:
Overhead squat- 4 x 3 (3 sec pause on first rep)

WOD: 3 min round clock
12 x hang power snatch (40/30)
10 x box jump
8 x push press
Max effort bar muscle up or burpee pull up

Rest 2 min
Repeat x 5

Session 1316
Strength/skill:
Max effort ring dips x 4
Or
4 x 10 assisted

WOD: for time
200m waiters carry (100m out 100m back) (22.5/15)
40 x kB sumo high pull (24/16)

200m single arm racked carry
30 x kB sumo high pull

200m double farmer carry
20 x kB sumo high pull

400m run
10 x kB sumo high pull

Session 1317

Strength/skill:
Bench press heavy 2

DB bench press 3x10

WOD: 3 rounds for time
15 x clean and jerk (50/35)

12 x bar facing burpee
9 x pull up

Session 1318

Front squat heavy 2

Back squat 1 x 20 60%

WOD: amrap 9 min
Wallball x 35
Double unders x 50

Session 1319

5th birthday WOD!

25 rounds for time
3 x thruster (40/30)
3 x bar over burpee
3 x pull up

Session 1320

2 rounds for time
200m run
10 x Db snatch left arm
200m run
10 x Db snatch right arm

Rest

2 rounds for time
15 x cluster (60/40)
5 x rope climb

Rest

If time allows
21/15/9

Burpee box jump
KB sumo high pull (24/16)

Session 1321

Strength/skill:
Strict press - heavy 3

WOD: 5 rounds for time
20 x deadball lunges
5 x man makers (22.5/15)
2 x muscle ups

Session 1322
Strength/skill:
Deadlift- heavy 3
*perform 4 sets of 2 heavy Db snatches each arm in between deadlift sets, focus on violent hip extension

WOD: 20 min clock
200 x double unders
100 x Kb swing (24/16)
80 x single arm Db push jerk (22.5/15)
60 x Db hang power clean

In remaining time amrap
15 x Db thruster
15 x box jump

Session 1323
Strength/skill:
3 position power clean (above knee, below knee, ground). Work to max

WOD - 17 min amrap
3 x power clean (80/55)
1 x round "gymcomp"
6 x power clean
1 x round of "gymcomp "

9 x power clean
1 x round of "gymcomp"

Etc......
*gymnastic complex - 3 x burpee, 5 x pull up, 7 x push up

Session 1324
Strength
Front squat- heavy 3

Back squat 1 x 20 @ 58.5%

WOD: 11 min ascending ladder x 2
Db box step overs (22.5/15)
Ttb

Session 1325
12 min partner amrap
Round for round
6 x Db snatch
6 x burpee

Rest 2

12 min partner amrap
Round for round
6 x Db hang clean and jerk
6 x burpee pull up

Rest 2

12 min partner amrap
Max cals bike or row
Swapping every minute

*Every 3 min both partners perform 10 goblet squats

Session 1326

3RFT
15 x DB power clean (22.5/15)
12 x DB front squat
9 x DB push press

Rest

12 min amrap
75 x double unders
100m farmers carry
30 x sit ups

Session 1327
Strength/skill:
Weighted dips - 5x5

WOD:
3 rounds for time
100 x walking lunges
50 x wallball

*starting with and every 4 min after 200m run

Session 1328

Strength/skill:
Sumo high pull - 5 x 5

*After each set perform 3 slam ball as hard as possible, think about throwing
ball through the ground

WOD: amrap 15 min
Box jump x 50
Turkish get up x 5 each arm (24/16)
Single Racked kB box step over x 10

Session 1329

Strength/skill:
Push press 5x5

WOD: for time
30/20/10
Plate snatch
Burpee pull up

Or

30 x plate snatch
9 x burpee muscle up
20 x plate snatch
6 x burpee muscle up
10 x plate snatch
3 x burpee muscle up

Session 1330

Strength/skill:
Front squat work to heavy 5

Back squat 1 x 20 @55%

WOD: 10 min ascending ladder x2
O/H lunge (40/30)
Hang power clean
30 x double unders (constant)

Session 1331

40 min strongman

WOD: partner Amrap 10 min

Partner A: 400m run
Partner B: amrap
5 x deadball push press
5 x burpee over deadball

5 x deadball squat

Session 1332

For time as 2 person team
200 x thruster (20/15)
150 x Db snatch (22.5/15)
100 x pull up
100 x hspu

Session 1333
Strength/skill:
Deadlift 7 x 2 @ 60% (speed focus)
In between sets perform a max effort broad jump double.

WOD: amrap 20min
15 x db hang squat clean (22.5/15)
12 x TTB
9 x renegade rows (no push up)
400m run

Session 1334

Strength/skill:
Standing DB chest pass to wall 5 x 3 hard and fast.

Bench press speed focus 8 x 3 @ 60% (60-90 sec rest)

WOD:
3 rounds for time
30 x hr push-up
20 x sumo high pull (60/40)
10 x S2O

E2MOM -10 x sit ups

Session 1335

Strength/skill:

Seated box jump x 20
Back squat 1 x 20 @ 50%

WOD: for max reps
1 min thruster (40/30)
1 min pull up
1 min bar facing burpee
1 min double under
Rest 1 min
Repeat x 4 rounds

Session 1336

4 rounds for time
400m run
6 x single arm Db thruster left (22.5/15)
6 x single arm Db thruster right
6 x left arm Db hang clean and jerk
6 x right arm Db hang clean and jerk

Rest

Amrap 15 min
50m deadball carry
1 x rope climb or peg board
50m racked Db carry
1 x rope climb or peg board

Session 1337

Strength/skill:
Deadlift - find heavy single

In between ramp up sets perform 3 x 8 bent over rows (a total of 3 sets, not 3 sets each rest)

WOD: amrap 12 min
Cluster from hang x 2 (60/40)
Front rack lunge x 4
Db snatch x 8 (22.5/15)

Session 1338
Strength/skill:
Weighted pull up 5/5/3/3/1/1

WOD: "filthy 50"
50 box-jumps
50 pull ups
50 kettlebell swings (24/16)
50 lunges
50 knees to elbows
50 push-presses (20/15)
50 wallballs
50 burpees
50 double-unders

Session 1339

Strength/skill:
Bench press- build to heavy single

Db bench 3 x 8-10

WOD: 10 - 1
Hspu
TTB
*after each round perform 100m farmer carry (22.5/15)

Session 1340

Strength/skill:
Front squat work to heavy single (10 min)
Back squat - 1 x 20 @

WOD: for time
21/15/9
Thruster (40/30)
Hang power clean

Into 400m run

Into
12/9/6
Thruster (50/35)
Pull up

Session 1341
20 min partner amrap
Round for round
5 x Db shoulder to overhead left arm
5 x Db S2O right arm
10 x med ball clean

Rest

20min clock
In a 1 min window
Partner A
10 x slam ball
Max effort wallballs

Swap every minute.
Workout is over when 200 wallballs are complete or time is up

Session 1342

3 rounds for time
40 x double unders
7 x power snatch (50/35)
3 x muscle up

Rest

Amrap 10 min
Ascending ladder x1

Burpee box jump over
Devil press (22.5/15)

Rest

Tabata hollow hold

Session 1343

Strength/skill:
Overhead squat- heavy 3 for the day

WOD: 6 min amrap
1 x rope climb
7 x TTB
9 x kB swing

Rest 2 min

6 min amrap
30 x plate thruster (20/15)
30 x sit ups
30 x kB sumo high pull

Rest 2 min

For time
2 x rope climb
14 x TTB
18 x kB swing
30 x plate thruster
30 x sit ups
30 x kB sumo high pull

Session 1344

Strength/skill:
Ring row 4 x max effort (feet elevated if possible)

WOD: amrap 20 min
30 x DB box step overs (22.5/15) (20inch for all)
15 x renegade rows
*100m sprint at start and every 4 minutes

Session 1345

Strength/skill:
Push press 5 x 3

WOD: 21/18/15/12/9/6
Power clean (40/30)
Push press
*10 lateral bar hops every break

Session 1346

Strength/skill:
Front squat 3 x 3
Back squat 1 x 20 @50%

WOD: amrap 10 min
8 x left arm DB lunges
12 x pull up
8 x right arm DB lunges
12 x push up

Rest 2 min

Amrap 5 min
Burpee pull up
*emom 3 x Db hang clean n jerk

Session 1347

Strongman 40min

WOD: partner WOD
Amrap 10 min
Partner A: 100m pinch grip farmer carry
Partner b: amrap
5 x renegade rows
10 x jumping lunges
15 x sit up

Session 1348

2 rounds for time
400m run
20 x back squat @55% of 1rm
10 x muscle up

Rest

3 rounds for time
21 x wallball
15 x chest to bar pull up
9 x clean and jerk (60/40)

Session 1349

Strength/skill:
Bench press 4x7

WOD: death by burpee box jump
*once fail to complete reps continue sequence from the same number with just box jumps till failure

Rest 2 min after last person

30 x air squat
800m run
30 x push up

Session 1350

Strength/skill:
Deadlift 4x7

WOD: amrap 20 min
Ascending ladder x 2
Db snatch each arm (22.5/15)
TTB
30 x double unders

Session 1351
Strength/skill:
Strict press 4 x 7

WOD: 2 rounds for time
30 x burpee
25 x kB swing (24/16)
20 x thruster (50/35)
15 x pull up

Session 1352

Strength/skill:
Front squat- 4 x 7 (leaving 2 in the tank)

WOD: starting a new round every 5 min x 25min

20 x wallball
400m run
2 x hang squat clean (80/55)

Session 1353

12 day of Xmas!
Last WOD for the year. We all know the drill, if your new to this ask the coach
how it works and have fun!

1- cluster (50/35)
2- front squat
3- hang power clean
4- push jerk
5- deadlift
6- bar over burpee
7- push up
8- wallballs
9- sit ups
10- TTB
11- thrusters
12- front rack lunges

Session 1354
Strength/skill:
Speed focus deadlifts 8 x 3 @ 60% (90 sec rest)

WOD: 18/15/12
Db snatch (22.5/15)
Pull up

Rest 2 min

9/6/3
Db snatch (32.5/22.5)
Bar muscle up
Deadball over shoulder (pick heavy weight)

Session 1355

Strength/skill:
Weighted dips - 5x5

WOD: 2 rounds for time
50 x ttb
50 x box jump
800m run

Session 1356
Strength/skill:
Squat clean work to heavy single

WOD: for time
50 x cluster (50/35)
*emom 5 burpees

Session 1357

For time
15 x power snatch (60/40)
30/20 cal bike
15 x power snatch

Rest

4 rounds for time
21 x wallball
18 x pull up
15 x Kb swing (24/16)
12 x hspu

Session 1358
Strength/skill:
Front squat - 3 x 3

Back squat (partials)
3 x 20
*go to full depth but don't lock out up top

WOD: amrap 14 min
400m run
30 x OH plate lunge (20/15)
30 x sit up

Session 1359

Strength/skill:
Pull up - 4 x max effort
Superset
Single arm Db row - 8 each arm

WOD: 90 sec on 1 min off
8 x deadlift (80/55)
5 x bar over burpee
Max renegade rows (no push up)

Repeat until

Session 1360

Strength/skill:
Bench press 1 rm

WOD:
1-10 clean and jerk (50/35)
2-20 push up

Session 1361
Strength/skill:
Find heavy complex - power clean/ hang squat clean/ front squat/ push jerk/ thruster

WOD: 3 rounds for time
35 x double Db snatch
35 x wallball

Session 1362

Strength/skill:
40 min strongman

WOD: 10 min partner amrap
Partner A: 200m run
Partner B: amrap
15 x wallball
Max burpees

*swap

Score is burpees

Session 1363

15/12/9
Power snatch (50/35)
Box jump

Rest

15/12/9
Hang squat clean
KTE
ring dip

Rest

15/12/9
Deadlift
Push press
Bar facing burpee

Session 1364

Strength/skill:
Front squat - work to heavy triple (first rep to have 3 sec pause at bottom)

WOD: 21/15/9/15/21
Thruster (30/20)
Pull up

Session 1365

Strength/skill:
Pendlay row - 5 x 5

WOD: 5 rounds for time

100 m Farmer carry (22.5/15)
100m DB front rack carry
400m run

Session 1366

Strength/skill:
Squat clean work to heavy double

WOD: amrap 18 min
15 x single OH Db lunges left arm (22.5/15)
15 x single Db hang clean and jerk left arm
15 x of Db lunge right arm
15 x Db hang clean and jerk right arm

E3mom - 1 round of Cindy

Session 1367

Strength
Oh squat 5x3

WOD: for time
50 x box jump
50 x sumo high pull (60/40)
50 x bar facing burpee

Session 1368
Partner wods

10 min amrap
Partner A - 100m dball carry
Partner B - amrap man makers

10 min amrap
Partner A - 100m farmer carry
Partner B - amrap burpee pull up

10 min amrap
Partner A - 200m run
Partner B - amrap over head plate lunges

Session 1369

3 rounds
30 x overhead squat (20/15)
30m overhead Db walk (22.5/15)

Rest

Amrap 7 min
15 x sit up
15 x KB swing (24/15)

Rest

If time allows

For time
1km row
Or
50/35 cal bike

Session 1370

Strength/skill:
Weighted pull - 5x5

WOD: 5 x 2 min rounds
30 x wall ball
Max effort ttb
1 min rest between rounds

Session 1371

Strength/skill:
Bench press - 5 x 5 paused bench press

WOD: 30/20/10
Alternating Db snatch (22.5/15)
Single arm OH Db box step overs

Session 1372
Strength/skill:
Squat snatch - work to a heavy single

WOD: "DT"
5 rounds for time
12 x deadlift (70/50)
9 x hang power clean
6 x push jerk

Session 1373

1rm squat

WOD: for time

30 x burpee muscle ups
Or
60 x burpee pull up
(10 min cap)

Session 1374

40 min strongman

WOD: 10 min partner amrap

5 x slamball burpee
3 x burpee
1 x slam ball

*you go I go

Session 1375

As pairs for time

40 x clean and jerks (80/55)
Row/bike/run

30 x clean and jerks
Row/bike/run

20 x clean and jerks
Row/bike/run

10 x clean and jerks
Row/bike/run

*choose either run 1km together/
Row 1.5kms swapping every minute
Or bike 80/55 cal swapping every minute

Session 1376

Strength/skill:
Strict press - 5x3 (3 sec eccentric)

WOD: 4 rounds
10 x kB clean to lunge left arm (24/16)
10 x kB clean to lunge right arm
20 x burpee

Session 1377

Strength/skill:
Thruster - 5/5/3/3

WOD: running clock
From 0-15min
3 rounds
40 x wall balls
30 x sit ups
20 x sumo high pull (40/30)

From 15-24min
Choose 1
    1.6k run
    100/70 cal bike
    2k row

*if you don't complete the 3 rounds in the 15 cap in part A go strait into part B

Session 1379

Strength/skill:
Power clean 5 x 2

WOD: 15 rounds for time

2 x bar muscle up
4 x Db power clean (22.5/15)
8 x push up

Session 1380

Squat

Amrap 10 min
Ttb x 12
Box jump x 24

100m sprint

Session 1381
40 min clock
In pairs complete

250 x Db clean and jerk
250 x pull up
250 x renegade row (no push up)

*both partners may work at the same time chipping away at the total swapping as needed.
*if all reps completed in 40 min cap, both partners amrap cals on bike or rower and burpees swapping every minute

Session 1382

Amrap 20 min
2 x muscle up
8 x kB swing (32/24)
16 x wallball

Rest

21/15/9
Power clean (60/40)
Front squat
Push jerk

Session 1383

Strength/skill:
Bench press - 8 x 3 @65-70% (speed focus) 90 sec rest

WOD: amrap 15 min
50 x double under
10 x sumo high pull (50/35)
200m run
10 x hang power clean

Session 1384

Strength/skill:
Ring dips- 10/8/6/4/2

WOD- rowing Barbara

5 rounds for time
20 x ring row (horizontal for RX)
30 x push up
40 x sit up
50 x air squat

3 min rest between rounds

Session 1385

Strength/skill:
In 10 min
Find heavy Complex - power clean/hang power clean/ strict press/ push press

Then
Emom 4 min
85% of above max

WOD: 6 rounds for time
6 x hspu
8 x c2b
6 x clean and jerk (70/50)

Session 1386
Strength-
Squats
2x1 -95
2x3 -9

WOD: amrap 10 min
Ascending x 2
Thruster (40/30)
Bar facing burpee

Session 1387

40 min strongman

WOD: amrap 10 min
Partner 1- 200m run
Partner 2- amrap cals bike/row

Swap

Session 1388

5 rounds for time
15 x wallball
15 x power clean (40/30)

Rest

10-1
Burpee
Pull up

Session 1389
Strength/skill:
Deadlift- 12 min to establish a 3rm

WOD: for time
1000m run
15 x box jump
10 x Db hang squat clean (22.5/15)

800m run
15 x box jump
20 x Db hang squat clean

400m run
15 x box jump
30 x Db hang squat clean

Session 1390
Strength/skill:
Bench press - 10/8/6/4/2

WOD-
In a 5 min window complete 7 rounds of "the chief" @ 50/35 then max effort burpees in remainder

Rest 3 min

In a 5 min window complete 5 rounds of "the chief" @70/50 then max effort burpees in remainder

*the chief is 3x power clean, 6 x push up, 9 x air squat.

Session 1391
Strength
Squatzzzz

WOD: amrap 10 min

Ascending ladder
Devils press
Box step up

Session 1392

21/15/9
Power clean (50/35)
Thruster

Rest

9-15-21
Double Db snatch (22.5/15)
HR push up
Ring dip

Session 1393
Strength/skill:
Thruster - 5/4/3/2/1

WOD: amrap 20 min
5 x squat clean (70/50)
5 x push jerk
400m run

Session 1394
Strength/skill:
Ring row 5 x 10-15

WOD: running clock
3 rounds
15 x kte
15 x kB swing (24/16)

Rest 2 min

3 rounds
15 x med ball cluster
50 x double under

Rest 2 min

1 round
45 x kte
45 x KB swing
45 x med ball cluster
150 x double under

Session 1395

Strength/skill:
Hang power snatch find 3rm

WOD: 10/8/6/4/2
Burpee pull up
Deadlift (120/85)
200m rum

Session 1396

Strength
Back squat
2x1 92%
5x2 88%

WOD: amrap 10 min

20 x Db lunge
30 x sit up

Session 1397
Partner WOD

Amrap 20 min
10 x ring row
8 x Db thruster
3 x deadball over shoulder

Round for round
*partner resting must hold Kb in rack

Rest

Amrap - 10 min
Partner 1- 200m run
Partner 2- Db burpee step ups
Swap

Session 1398

For time

In pairs
100 x clean and jerk (50/35)
100 x bar muscle up
200 x wallball
100 x hspu
100 x sumo high pull

Divide reps as needed

Session 1399
Strength/skill:
Pendlay row - 5x5

WOD: amrap 15 min
25 x power snatch (40/30)
25 x box jump
25 x ttb

Session 1400

Strength/skill:
2 Pos power clean x 5 (above knee, ground)

WOD: 10 x complex
5 x deadlift (70/45)
4 x front squat
3 x hang power clean
2 x push press
1 x thruster
*if bar is let go during complex rep will not count, you may let go between reps

Session 1401

Strength/skill:
Bench press 3x10 ahap
Superset
Kneeling dball chest pass to wall x5

WOD: start a new round every 4 min x 5 rounds
30 x KB sumo Hugh pull (24/16)
10 x KB clean and jerk each arm
15 x renegade rows (22.5/15)

Session 1402

Strength/skill

Back 7x3 87%

WOD amrap 10 min
100m farmer walk (22.5/15)
10 x Db thruster
8 x pull up

Session 1403

40 min strongman

WOD: amrap 10 min
Partner 1 - run 200m
Partner 2 - amrap Cindy
*swap when runner returns

Session 1404
Amrap 11 min
7 x ttb
8 x Db lunge (22.5/15)
7 x Db push press

Rest

2 rounds for time
30 x back squat (60/40)
20 x push up
10 x box jump

*no rack

Session 1405

Strength/skill:
Hang squat clean - 3/3/2/1/1
Superset
Seated box jump x 2

WOD: for time
50 x kb snatch left arm (24/16)
30 x deadball over shoulder
50 x kb snatch right

30 x burpee

Session 1406
Strength/skill:
Deadlift 5 x 5

WOD: amrap 4 min
60 x double unders
6 x muscle ups
Max effort Db box step overs in remainder(22.5/15)

Rest 1 min repeat x 3 rounds

Session 1407

Strength/skill:
Weighted pull up - 5x5

WOD: 3 rounds for time
21 x Hspu
18 x sumo high pull (50/35)
15 x shoulder to overhead
12 x hang power clean

Session 1408

In teams amrap 40 min

200 cal bike/row (swapping every 30sec)
50 synchro lunges
50 synchro jumping lunges
200 med ball cleans

Session 1409

For time as a two person team
100 x push jerk (60/40)

90 x ghd sit ups or KTE
80 x push ups
70 x kB swing (32/24)
60 x bar facing burpee
50 x front squat (60/40)
40 x rope climb

Divide reps as needed working down the list.

Session 1410

Strength/skill:
Weighted dip 5 x 5
Or 5 x 10 banded

WOD: 3 rounds for time
30 x box jump
30 x sit ups
30 x hang squat clean (30/25)
200m run

Session 1411
Strength/skill:
Sumo high pull 3x3 ahap

WOD: for time
30 x clean and jerk (40/30)
20 x front rack lunges
30 x burpee pull up
20 x front rack lunge
30 x clean and jerk

Session 1412

Strength/skill:
Bench press- 7 x 1
Superset
Dball push press to wall x 3

WOD : 21/15/9
Ttb

Db hang power clean (22.5/15)
Plate snatch (20/15)

Session 1413

40 min strongman prac

WOD: partner amrap 10 min
40 x Plate snatch
20 x burpee to plate
10 x overhead plate lunge
*all movements synchro

Session 1414

3 rounds for time
400m run
20 x pull ups

Amrap 15 min
5 x man makers (22.5/15)
10 x deadlift (100/70)
15 x HR push ups

Session 1415
Strength/skill:
3 x Strict press + 5 x push press: 4 sets

WOD: for time
100 thrusters (40/30)
*every break perform 5 hang power cleans and 5 burpees

Session 1416

Strength/skill:
O/h squat - 3 x 5

WOD: for time
50 x ttb
5 x dball squat clean (ahap)
50 x kB swing
4 x dball squat clean
50 x sit ups
3 x dball squat clean
50 x hollow rocks
2 x dball squat clean
50 x v -ups
1 x dball squat clean

Session 1417

Strength/skill:
Clean and jerk - find heavy double

WOD: 10 rounds for time
1 x clean and jerk (80/55)
5 x weighted pull-up (10/7.5)
10 x box jump

10 min amrap
30 x oh lunges (15 each arm)
20 x hr push ups
10 x Db snatch

Session 1418
Hero WOD "glen"
30 x clean and jerk (60/40)
1.6km run
10 x rope climb
1.6km run
100 x burpee

Session 1419

Strength/skill:

Bench press - 10/5/10/5/10/5
(Goal is to increase each wave by at least 2.5kg)
*after each set of 5 perform 3 plyo push ups

WOD: 18 min running clock
800m run
5 DB Turkish get ups on each side (22.5/15)
In remainder of time AMRAP
3 x burpee muscle up
6 x Db push jerk each arm
12 x Db snatch

Session 1420
Strength/skill:
Paused front squat 5x2 (3sec pause)

WOD: for time
75 x racked kb lunge (24/16)
50 x kb clean and jerk
25 x racked kb box step up

Emom - 5 x kb swing

Session 1421

Strength/skill:
5 x max effort pull ups

WOD: 4 rounds for time
80 x double unders
10 x renegade rows (22.5/15)
80 x double unders
10 x sumo high pull (60/40)

Session 1422

Squats 4x8 @75%

Accessory-
Sit squat
3x10 weighted

WOD: amrap 10 min
Thruster x 8 (40/30)
Bar da ing burpee

Session 1423

Team WOD: amrap 40 min
In teams 1 rep at a time each
80 wallballs
80 sit ups
80 burpees
80 dball cleans
200m suitcase carry (22.5/15)

Session 1424

For time
800m run
30 x clean and jerk (50/35)
10 x rope climb
800m run
25 x clean and jerk
8 x rope climb
800m run
20 x clean and jerk
6 x rope climb
800 m run

Session 1425

Strength/skill:
Push press- 7/5/5/3/3

WOD: amrap 14 min
7 x muscle up

14 x Db snatch (22.5/15)
21 x ttb

Session 1426

Strength/skill:
Hang power clean 5 x 2

WOD: for time
150 x wallballs
Emom- 5 x box jumps

Session 1427

Strength/skill:
Bench press - 6 x 2
*3 double kneeling chest pass to wall with deadball after each set. Explosive as possible.

WOD: 4 x 5 min rounds
400m run
30 x DB push jerk (15/10)
Max effort deadball cleans (go heavy)
1 min rest

Session 1428

Strength
Squat- 3x 10 @ 70%

Accessory -
Bulgarian split squat each leg
1 x 12 bw
1 x 10 with dbs
1 x 8 with heavier dbs

WOD: amrap 10 min
15 x db hang squat clean

15 x burpee over Db

Session 1428

40 min of Strongman

WOD: amrap 10 min with partner

100 single arm DB thruster (22.5/15)
100 lateral box step ups

(1 person working at a time, divide reps as neede)

Session 1430

4 rounds for time
4 x power clean (80/55)
4 x front squat
4 x shoulder to overhead

Rest

21/15/9
hang power snatch (40/30)
*7 muscle ups after each round

Session 1431

Strength/skill:
Sumo deadlifts 5x5

WOD: amrap 15 min
40 x Kb swing (24/16)
40 x Burpee pull up

Session 1432

Strength/skill:
Ring dips 5 x max effort
Or

5 x 10 assisted

WOD: for time
100 x squat
4 x rope climb
75 x squat
3 x rope climb
50 x squat
2 x rope climb
25 x squat
1 x rope climb

Session 1433
Strength/skill:
Power clean + hang power clean 8 sets (90 sec rest)

WOD: 4 rounds for time
12 x hang power clean and strict press (40/30)
200m run
12 x TTB
200m run

Session 1434

Swyatzzzz

WOD: amrap 10 min
20 x Db snatch
10 x burpee box jump

Session 1435

4 rounds for time
15 x wallball
12 x chest to bar
9 x single arm DB push press (27.5/20)

Rest

7 rounds for time

35 x double under
7 x KB swing (32/24)
5 x ring dip

Session 1436

Strength/skill:
Bench press- 5x3
Superset
Dball push press for height to wall x3

WOD: for time
3 rounds of Cindy
15 x hang cluster (50/35)
2 rounds of Cindy
10 x hang cluster
1 round of Cindy
5 x hang cluster

Session 1437

Strength/skill:
Sumo high pull - 5 x 5
*3 x seated box jump after each set

WOD- 3 Rounds for time

Lateral bar hop x 50
Deadlift x 12 (100/70)
400m run
100m waiter carry (22.5/15. 50 out/50 back)

Session 1438
Strength/skill:
Pull up 10/10/7/7/5/5 (use weight or bands to get desired rep range)

WOD:
40 x DB hang clean and jerk (22.5/15)

40 x HR push up
20 x ttb
10 x bar muscle up
20 x ttb
40 x HR push up
40 x DB hang clean and jerk

Session 1439
Strength/skill:
Back squat - 3x10 @ 65% ?

Accessory
Bulgarian split squat 3x12

WOD: 10-1
Dball slam
Dball lunges

Session 1440
In teams amrap 40 min
200 cal bike/row swapping every 30sec
100 burpees (1 at a time)
50 synchro plate snatches

Session 1441

3 rounds for time
75 x double unders
20 x box step ups with Db overhead (15/10) (10 right arm,10 left arm)

Rest

"Grace"
30 x clean and jerk (60/40)

Rest

Tabata
Sit up
Hanging knee raise

Session 1442

Strength/skill:
Push jerk 3/1/3/1/3/1

WOD: 10 rounds
8 x DB snatch
7 x box jump
6 x burpee pull up
(40 sec work/ 20 sec rest)

Session 1443
Strength/skill:
Deadlift - work up to 1 set of 5 @ 80%

WOD: amrap 20min
Hspu x 9
Ttb x 5
KB swing x 18 (24/16)
Ttb x5
Double under x 36

Session 1444

Strength/skill:
Hang power snatch - 2rm

WOD:
60 x wallball
Into
3 rounds
24 x front rack lunges (40/30)
12 x clean and jerk
Into
30 x wallball

Session 1445

Strength/skill:
Bench press 5x5 (no bounce)
Superset
Wall ball push press (use dball)

WOD: for time
50 x renegade rows (22.5/15)
Emom -8 sit ups

Session 1446

Strength/skill:
Strongman 30-40 min

WOD: 10 min partner amrap
Partner a - 200m run
Partner b - amrap of 5 slam ball, 7 burpee over ball, 5 dball thruster

Swap when partner a returns from run

Session 1447

For time
20 x back squat (80/55)
1.6km run
20 x back squat

Rest

For time
50 x burpee box jump

Session 1448

Strength/skill:
Strict press 5/4/3/5/4/3

WOD- for time and load
80 x deadball push press (pick own load)
*(Every break perform 5 x ttb and 5 x Db hang power clean 22.5/15)

Session 1449

Strength/skill:
Cluster - 3/3/2/2/1/1

WOD:
Tabata
kb snatch
Goblet lunge

Rest 2 min

Tabata
Box jump
Cluster (40/30)

Session 1450

Strength/skill:
Weighted pull-ups 5/5/3/3/1/1

WOD: Bradley
100m sprint
10 x pull up
100m sprint
10 x burpee
Rest 30 sec

Session 1451

Strength/skill:
Back squat 5x2 (4,3,x,0)

WOD:
20/18/16/14/12/10
Wallball
SIingle arm DB hang clean + jerk

Session 1452

Team WOD:
In teams of 3

Amrap 40 min
300 cal bike/row (swapping every 30 sec)
400 m walk with - deadball and 3 kbs
(Deadball can carry however you like, person with 2 kbs must farmer carry, person with 1 kb must rack carry. Swap as needed)

Session 1453

3 rounds
400m run
21 x KB swing (24/16)
2 x rope climb

Rest

21 x push press (40/30)
7 x bar muscle up
15 x push press
7 x bar muscle up
9 x push press
7 x bar muscle up

Session 1454

Strength/skill:
Deadlift - 3 x 3 ahap (reset each rep)

WOD: 20 min clock
Min 1 - amrap wallball
Min 2 - amrap hang power clean (60/40)
Min 3 - amrap bar facing burpee
Min 4 - plank
Min 5 rest
Repeat x 4
(round 4 attempt a 2min plank)

Session 1455

Strength/skill:
Bench press - 5/4/3/5/4/3

WOD: for time
50 x sit ups
10 x devils press (22.5/15)
40 x sit ups
8 x devils press
30 x sit ups
6 x devils press
20 x sit ups
4 x devils press
10 x sit ups
2 x devils press

Session 1456
Strength/skill:
Overhead squat - 5 x 3 (3,3,x,0)

WOD: 4 rounds
50 x double unders
15 x ttb
12 x thruster (45/32.5)

Session 1457

Strength
3 position clean clean
Above knee/ below knee/ ground
Find heavy

WOD:
21/15/9
DB deadlift
DB push jerk

Into

20 burpee muscle ups
Or
40 burpee pull ups

Session 1458

Strength/skill:
Strongman

WOD: amrap 10 min with partner
Partner Med ball sit ups

Emom - Both partners perform 10 med ball cleans

Session 1459

3rft

400m run
15 x ttb
9 x power snatch

Rest

Amrap 15 min
15 x burpee pull up
15 x thruster (40/30)
45 x double under

Session 1460

Strength/skill:
Overhead lunges - 5 x 10 (5 each leg)

WOD: 2 rounds for time
40 x box jump
30 x DB snatch (22.5/15)
20 x DB box step overs

Session 1461

Strength/skill:
Sumo high pull 5 x 5

WOD: amrap 20 min
50 x HR push ups
5 x Turkish get up left arm (24/16)
50 x KB swing

50 x HR push ups
5 x Turkish get up right arm
50 x KB swing

Session 1462
Emom
5 front squats x 3 rounds start at 30% increase 10%

Strength/skill :
Push jerk 3/3/2/2/1/1

WOD: 15/12/9/12/15
Pull up
Hang clean and jerk (50/35)

Session 1463

Skill: 30 min strongman

WOD: with a partner
10 min amrap
1 for 1 burpees
Emom - 8 DB snatch

Session 1464

5 rounds for time

20 x medball clean
10 x strict press (40/30)
2 x rope climb

Rest

For time
30 x Kb swing (28/20)
30/20 cal bike
30 x lunge

Session 1465
Strength/skill:
Overhead squat - 5 x 5

WOD- ascending ladder 18 min
1 x bear complex (50/35) (increase x1)
50 x double under (remains same)

Session 1466

Strength/skill:
Bench press - 5 x 3

WOD - 50/80 intervals x 10 rounds

Ttb x 5
Burpee x 8
Dball to shoulder x max effort

Session 1467
Strength/skill:
Weighted ring dips 5x5

WOD- 20 Rounds
5 x wallball
1 x man maker (22.5/15)

Session 1468

Strength/skill:

Power clean - 3/2/1/1/2

WOD:
15 x cluster (40/30)
21 x Pull ups

12 x cluster (50/35)
15 x C2B

9 x cluster (60/40)
9 x bar muscle up

Session 1469

30 min partner amrap

100 x burpee pull up
100 x OH plate lunges
100 x med ball sit ups
100 x med ball clean

(Swap every 5 reps)

Session 1470

3 rounds for time
100m farmer carry (22.5/15)
12 x DB thrusters

Rest

5 rounds for time
400m run
12 x DB burpee deadlifts
4 x renegade rows

Session 1471

Strength/skill:

Front squat 1rm

WOD: death by wallball (x2)

Session 1472

Strength/skill:
Weighted pull up - 5 x 5

WOD- for time
150 x double under
4 x hang power clean (80/55)
50 x burpee
3 x hang power clean
100 x box jump
2 x hang power clean
50 x burpee
1 x hang power clean
150 x double under

Session 1473

Strength/skill:
Strict press 5/5/5
Push press 3/3/3

WOD: amrap 9 min
TTB x 8
DB snatch x 12 (22.5/15)

Session 1474
Strength/skill:
Clean and jerk - 3/2/2/2/1

WOD- in 1 min
25 air squat
Amrap c+j (70/50)
Rest 1 min
Repeat x 8

Session 1475

Strength/skill:
30 min practicing strongman tools

WOD: as pairs
Amrap 10 min
7 x burpee
14 x kB swing
(Wile one partner is doing rounds other partner clocks up cals on rower/bike.
Swap every minute)

Session 1476

3 rounds for time
15 x deadlift (70/50)
12 x hang power clean
9 x push jerk

Rest

3 rounds for time
10 x HSPU
10 x hang squat clean (70/50)

Session 1477

Strength/skill
Front squat waves 3/2/1
90/92.5/95%
92.5/95.97.5%

WOD: 2 rounds for time
25 x TTB
50 x O/H lunges w/ plate (20/15)

Session 1478
Strength/skill:
Bench press - 7 x 2 (2 sec pause on chest)

WOD: 7 min ascending ladder (+1)
DB snatch left arm
DB push press left arm
DB snatch right arm
DB push press right arm

Session 1479
Strength/skill:
Overhead squat- 5x5

WOD - 13 min clock
3 rounds
20 x box jump
10 x DB burpee box step up (22.5/15)

Amrap Man makers in remainder

Session 1480
Strength/skill:
Power clean + hang power clean + push jerk (1+2+1) x 3

WOD:
9 x clean and jerk (80/55)
5 rounds of Cindy
6 x clean and jerk
5 rounds of Cindy
3 x clean and jerk
5 rounds of Cindy

Session 1481

Partner WOD

4 rounds for time
30 x synchro bar facing burpees
20 x synchro TTB

10 x synchro deadlifts (100/70)
200m partner farmer carry (22.5/16)

Session 1482

For time:
10 x dead ball clean*
11 x muscle up
100 x double under
11 x muscle up
10 x dead ball clean
(* pick a ball that is heavy enough that is challenging but won't compromise form)

Rest

For time
50 x HR push ups
50 x thrusters (30/20)

Session 1483
Strength/skill:
Strict press - 5x5

WOD: 10-1
Pull up
Sumo high pull (50/35)
*25 double unders after each round

Session 1484

Strength/skill:
Hang power snatch - heavy single

WOD: 2 rounds for time
40 x KB clean and jerk (24/16)
30 x box jump
20 x push up

Session 1485

Deadlift 1rm

WOD: amrap 7 min
5 x front squat
5 x push press
5 x thruster
5 x bar facing buried

Session 1486

Partner WOD

Amrap 10 min
50 x double under
10 x deadball ground to overhead

Rest 5 min

Amrap 10 min
18 x jumping lunge
10 cal bike or row

Rest 5 min

Amrap 10 min
10 x ring row
8 x plate thruster (20/15)

One partner working for 1 minute at a time

Session 1487
Amrap 5 min
5 x burpee
5 x muscle up

Rest

4 rounds for time

10 x power snatch (40/30)
15 x push jerk
10 x renegade rows (22.5/15)

Session 1488

Strength/skill:
Front squat waves -3/2/1
85/87.5/90%
87.5/90/92.5%

WOD: 5 rounds for time
Wallball x 20
DB Racked box step ups x 8 (15/10)

Session 1489

Strength/skill:
Squat clean 3/3/2/2

WOD: 13 min running clock
120 sit ups
Then amrap in remainder
15x Hspu
12x DB hang clean and jerk (22.5/15)
15 X KB Sumo high pull (24/16)

Session 1490
Strength/Skill
Bench press- 5 x 5

WOD: amrap 9 min
Ascending ladder
Burpee box jump (increase x 3)
Double under x 25 every round

Session 1491
Strength:
Strict press - 5/3/1/5/3/1

WOD: amrap 7 min
40 x double unders
12 x Db push press

Rest 3 min

Amrap 5 min
30 x double unders
6 x renegade row *no push up

Strength:

Front squat -
20 reps
1 minute rest
10 reps
30 sec rest
5 reps
30 sec rest
5 reps

WOD: for time
30 x sumo high pull (20/15)
30 x front squat
30 x hang squat clean
30 x power snatch
30 x overhead squat

Emom - 5 x burpees

Session 1492

Strength-
Deadlift 5 x 5

WOD: 21/15/9
Back squat (60/40)

Push jerk
*2 x man maker after each round

Session 1493

Strength:
Clean and jerk - find 2rm

WOD: amrap 20 min
50 x sit up
30 x Db snatch
50 x burpee
30 x single Db clean and jerk

Session 1494
Strength endurance:
Accumulate 100 push ups in as little sets as possible.

WOD: for time
1.6km farmer carry
Every time you have to break perform 5 thrusters.

Session 1495
Strength:
Bent over row- 7/7/5/5/3/3

WOD: 5 rounds for time
15 x push jerk (50/35)
15 x hang power clean
40 x double unders

Session 1496
Strength:

Front squat -
20 reps
1 minute rest
10 reps
30 sec rest

5 reps
30 sec rest
5 reps

WOD: amrap 12 min
35 x medball clean
8 x devil press

Session 1497

For time

1 round
150 x double unders
30 x high pull (40/30)
30 x burpees
Into
2 rounds
75 x double unders
15 x sumo high pull
15 x burpee
Into
3 rounds
50 x double unders
10 x sumo high pull
10 x burpee

Session 1498

Strength-
Strict press - 7/7/5/5/3/3

WOD:
5 x 3 min amraps

2 x renegade row
4x power clean (40/30)
6 x sit up

Rest 1 min Between amraps

Session 1499

Strength:
bent over row 5 x 5

WOD: for time
300 x walking lunge
EMOM - 5 x wallball

Session 1500
For time

1.6km run
Into
3 rounds
30 x Db snatch
30 x sit up
30 x strict press (30/20)
Into
1.6k run

Session 1501

Strength:
Hang squat clean - 5x3 *touch and go

WOD: running clock
EMOM x 5 min
5 x thruster (20/15)
5 x burpee
Strait into
EMOM X 5 min
7 x thruster
7 x burpee
Strait into
EMOM X 5 min
9 x thruster
9 x burpee

Session 1502
Front squat -
20 reps
1 minute rest
10 reps
30 sec rest
5 reps
30 sec rest
5 reps

WOD: for time
30 x Turkish get up
Emom - 7 x KB swings

Session 1503

20 rounds for time
1 x deadlift (120/85)
5 x bar over burpees
15 x double unders

Accessories:
Hollow rock -
30 seconds on 30 seconds off x 7

Session 1504
Strength- work up to a power clean 2rm. Then do 3 further sets of 2 at 90% of 2rm

WOD:
50 x sit ups
50 x push ups
50 x sit ups
50 x squats
50 x sit ups
50 x lunges
50 x sit ups

Session 1505

Strength-
bent over row - 7 x 3

WOD: ascending 12 min ladder
1 x renegade row
1 x double Db snatch

2 x renegade row
2 x double Db snatch

3 x renegade row
3 x double Db snatch

Etc.........

Session 1506
Strength-
Push press 5x5

WOD: 5 rounds for time
30 x wallball
5 x cluster (70/47.5)

Session 1507

3 rounds For time
800m run
15 x deadlift (100/70)
15 x Db push press

Accessories:
Hollow rocks - accumulate 75
Plank - accumulate 5 min

Session 1508
Strength-
bent over rows 5x5
After last set drop weight and do 1 set of 20

WOD:
21/15/9
Thruster (30/20)

Push up

Rest 3 min

15/12/9
Thruster (40/30)
Bar over burpee

Rest 3 min

9/6/3
Thruster (60/40)
Renegade row

Session 1509

Strength -
Work up to 80-85% of your clean and jerk

Then set a clock for 30 min and perform 1 clean and jerk every minute on the minute.

Session 1510
For time:

100 x double unders
30 x hang power snatch (40/30)
8 x Turkish gets ups

75 x double unders
20 x hang power snatch
6 x Turkish get up

50 x double unders
10 x hang power snatch
4 x Turkish get up

25 x double unders
5 x hang power snatch
2 x Turkish get up

Session 1511
Strength -
Deadlift - 3x5

WOD:
For time
50 x thruster (50/35)
50 x Db snatch
*emom 5 x burpees

Session 1512
Skill: 20 min of handstand practice

WOD: run bike or row for 30 min

Session 1513

Strength-
Strict press 7 x 3

WOD: 21/15/9
Push press (50/35)
Hang power clean
Push up

Session 1514

Strength
Bent over row 5x5

WOD: 3 min window
30 x wallball
10 x Db snatch
Max effort jumping lunge

Rest 1 min repeat x 6 rounds

Session 1515

For time:

20 x clean and jerk (60/40)
50 x bar facing burpee
20 x clean and jerk

Accessories:
Hollow rocks 5 x 15
Plank 3 x 1-2 min

Session 1516
Strength:
Deadlift- 3 x 5

WOD: amrap 12 min
18 x Kb sumo high pull
100m sprint
18 x Kb snatch
100m sprint

Session 1517
Strength-
Squat clean + 4 front squats
5 sets

WOD: 3 rounds for time
8 x Db hang power clean
10 x Db push press
12 x lunge with racked dbs

Accessories-
3 x max effort banana split

Session 1518

Strength -
Strict press 5 x 3
Bent over row 5 x 3

WOD:
30/20/10
kB swing
Sit ups

Rest 2 min

10/20/30
kB swing
Push up

Session 1519
For time
65 x wallball
75 x double under
10 x front squat (80/55)
800 m run
10 x front squat
65 x double under
75 x wallball

Session 1520

Strength-
clean and jerk 1rm

E3mom x 5 rounds - 1 clean and jerk @ 90% of above 1rm

WOD: amrap 15 min
75 x hang power clean (30/20)
50 x push press
25 x hang power snatch
*emom - 4 burpees

Session 1521
Strength- hang power clean 2rm

WOD-
21 x deadlift (100/70)
3 x Turkish get up
15 x deadlift
5 x Turkish get up
9 x deadlift
7 x Turkish get up

Session 1522

Strength
Bent over row 5 x 5
And/or
Pull ups (if possible)

WOD: for time
50 x overhead plate lunge (20/15)
10 x renegade row
40 x O/h lunge
8 x renegade row
30 x O/h plate lunge
6 x renegade row
20 x O/h plate lunge
4x renegade row
10 x O/h plate lunge
2 x renegade row

Session 1523

5 rft
5 x power clean (60/40)
10 x front squat
5 x push jerk
15 x burpee

Rest 90 sec between rounds

Session 1524

Strength
Power snatch - 5 x 2

WOD:
30 x double Db clean and jerk

3 min rest

50 push-ups for time

2 min rest

30 x Double Db hang snatch

Session 1525
15-1
Wallball
Sit up
*1 x bear complex after every round

Session 1526

Strength/skill:
Deadlift 3x5

WOD: Emom (every minute on the minute)
1 x Db deadlift
1 x Db hang power clean
20 x double under

*increase Db movements x 1 each minute.
Continue in this fashion untill you can't beat the clock.

Session 1527

Strength
Bent over row - 5 x 5

30/20/10
Front rack lunge (50/35)
Single arm push press

2 min window
200m sprint
15 x sir squat
Max effort cluster in remainder (50/35)

Rest 1 min
Repeat x 5 rounds

Session 1528

3 rounds for time
12 x hang power clean (60/40)
12 x devils press

Rest

20 Turkish get ups for time

Session 1529
Strength
Sumo high pull - 5 x 5

WOD:
5 rounds for time
400m run with wallball
200m farmer carry

Session 1530

Amrap 16 min

50 x Db hang snatch
100 x jumping lunge
150 x bar over burpees

*every 2 minutes on the minute perform 4 x deadlifts @ (100/70)

Session 1531

Strength/
20 min to work up to a power clean and strict press

WOD: 3 rounds for time
12 x barbell hang squat clean (60/40)
15 x Db push jerk

Rest 5 min

For time
100 x sit ups
Emom - 15 second plank

Session 1532

Amrap 9 min
12 x Db snatch
24 x push up

Rest 3 min
Into

3 rounds for time
15 x kB swing
15 x burpee

Session 1533

Strength/skill:
Back squat 5 x 5 @80%
Split squat 3 x 10 w/dbs

WOD: amrap 7 min
8 x Box jump
8 x hang power clean (50/35)
8 x ttb

Session 1534

20 min partner amrap
Partner A - 400m run
Partner B -
12 x kB lunge
6 x deadball over shoulder
12 x kB push jerk

Rest 5 min

Amrap 10min
Partner A - 100m farmer carry
Partner B -
8 x burpee
16 x wallball

Session 1535

5 rounds for time
12 x hspu
6 x power clean (70/47.5)

Rest

4 rounds for time
25 x sit up
15 x kB swing
5 x ring muscle up

Session 1536
Strength/skill:

Bench press - 5 x 3

WOD: 3 rounds for time
12 x Db cluster (22.5/15)
12 x renegade row
*1 min rest between rounds

Session 1537
Strength/skill:
Turkish get up - 15 min to find a heavy

WOD: for time
50 x Db snatch (22.5/15)
30 x burpee box jump
10 x single Db box step up
800m run
10 x single Db step up
30 x burpee box jump
50 x Db snatch

Session 1538
Strength/skill:
Hang squat clean/ hang power clean - 5 x 1 + 2

WOD: amrap 12 min
1 x Clean and jerk (50/35)
5 x pull up
10 x push up

*increase c+j x 1 each round

Session 1539

Strength/skill:
Back squat - 3 x 5 @ 70%*
Split squat - 3 x 10 unweighted
*deload - don't go heavier wade

WOD: 3 rounds for time
15 x thruster (40/30)

15 x ttb
400m run

Session 1540

Strongman

WOD: amrap 8 min
8 x Db hang clean and jerk
6 x wallball
4 x burpee pull up

Session 1541

21 x hspu
5 x rope climb
15 x hspu
3 x rope climb
9 x hspu
1 x rope climb

Rest

12 min ascending ladder
10 x air squat
10 x push up
1 x power snatch (50/35)

Increase squat and push ups x 2
Snatch remains @ 1

Session 1542
Strength/skill:
Pull up - 4 x max effort sets
Or
Accumulate 10-15 slow negative reps

WOD: 5 rounds for time
60 x double unders

5 x deadlift(60/40)
4 x hang power clean
3 x front squat
2 x push press
1 x push jerk

Rest 1 min

Session 1543

Strength/skill:
Strict press - 5 x 5

WOD: 21/15/9/15/21
Burpee
Kte

Session 1544
Strength/skill:
Back squat 4 x 8 @75%
Bulgarian split squat - 3 x 8 w/dbs

WOD:
amrap 8 min of Wallballs
Emom - 8 x box jump

Session 1545

40 min amrap

Partner WOD

40 x cal bike or row
30 x synchro bar facing burpees
20 x synchro TTB
10 x partner deadlifts
200m partner farmer carry (22.5/16)

Session 1546

2 rounds for time
20 x wallball
10 x power snatch (40/30)
20 x wallball
10 x clean and jerk
20 x wallball
10 x overhead squat
20 x wallball
10 x hang power clean

Session 1547
Strength/skill:
Sumo high pull - 5 x 3

WOD: 3 min window
20 x air squat
20 x push up
20 x sit up
Max effort Single Db hang clean & jerk (22.5/15
*if fail to get to Db reduce all reps x 5 h

Session 1548

Strength/skill:
Pendlay row - 5 x 3

WOD: 20 min ascending ladder
2 x renegade row *no push up (22.5/15)
2 x ttb
Increase x 2
*every 4 min perform 4 x Turkish get up

Session 1549

Strength/skill:
Close grip Bench press - 5 x 5

WOD: 8 rounds for time
30 x double unders
8 x push press (40/30)
3 x bar muscle up

Session 1550

Strength
Back squat 3 x 10 @70%
Split squat 3 x 15 each leg

WOD: amrap 10 min
20 x O/h single DB lunge (22.5/15)
5 x hang power clean (70/47.5)
10 x bar facing burpees

Session 1551

40min strongman

WOD: amrap 8 min
1 x deadball over bar
1 x man maker
*increase deadball x 1 each round

Session 1552

3 rounds for time
50 x double unders
15 x front squat (50/35)
9 x hspu

Rest

Amrap 15 min
10 x burpee to target
12 x Db* front rack box step over (22.5/15)

2 x rope climb
*1 DB

Session 1553

Strength/skill:
Power clean + hang power clean
Work to heavy

WOD: amrap 12 min
8 x pull up
12 x box jump
1 x deadlift (140/100)
*increase deadlift x 1 each round

Session 1554

Strength/skill:
Elevated feet ring rows 5 x 10-15

WOD: for time
50/40/30/20/10
kB swing (24/16)
Sit up
*100m front rack carry after each round

Session 1555

Strength/skill:
Hang power snatch - 5 x 2

WOD: 3 rounds for time
12 x double DB Hang snatch (22.5/15)
12 x burpee over DB
400m run

Session 1556
Strength
Back squat 4x8 @ 70%

Bulgarian split squat 3 x 12 each leg

WOD: amrap 10 min
30 x wallball
1 x clean and jerk (80/55)
*increase c&j x 1 each round

Session 1557
Amrap 20 min
Partner 1- 20/15 cals
Partner 2 - amrap of Cindy

Rest 10 min

Amrap 20 min
Partner 1 - 20/15 cals
Partner 2 - amrap
5 x Db thruster, 5 x ttb, 5 x renegade row

Session 1558

Amrap 13 min
25 x deadlift (100/70)
25 x wallball
25 x hspu

Rest

3 rounds for time
50 x double under
15 x knees to elbow
15 x push jerk (50/35)

Session 1559
Strength/skill:
Accumulate 3 min in l-sit
Accumulate 3 min in at top of dip

WOD: amrap 25 min

800m run
200m overhead plate carry (20/15)
100m farmer carry (22.5/15)
30 x box jump

Session 1560
Strength/skill:
Pendlay row - 4 x 6 (3 sec eccentric)

WOD: for time
30 x man maker (50/35)
Every break perform 2 x Turkish get up (22.5/15)

Session 1561
Strength/skill:
Push press + push jerk 5 x (2+3)

WOD: for time
100 x doburpeeuble unders
40 x burpee pull up
20 x clean and jerk (60/40)

Session 1562
Strength/skill:
Back squat - 3 x 10 @60%
Bulgarian split squat - 3 x 10 each leg (no weight)

WOD: amrap 8 min
30 x wallball
20 x ttb
10 x Db snatch (22.5/15)

Session 1563
40 min strongman

WOD: amrap 8 min
12 x alternating DB Clean and jerk

18 x sit up

Session 1564
3 rounds for time
15 x power snatch (40/30)
10 x bar facing burpees

Rest

3 rounds for time
21 x thruster (40/30)
15 x hang power clean
9 x hspu

Session 1565
Strength/skill:
Back rack lunges- 4 x 6 each leg

WOD: amrap 8 min
8 x Db box step overs (22.5/15)
12 x pull up

Rest 3 min

Amrap 5 min
3 x Sumo high pull 60/40
6 x box jump
9 x late bar hops

Session 1566
Strength/skill:
Ring dips - 10/10/8/8/6/6
*add weight to achieve reps

WOD: 5 rounds for time
25 x wallball
50 x double under
25 x kB swing (24/16)
*rest 1 min after each round

Session 1567
Strength/skill:
Bench press- 3 rm then
2x2 @95% of above

WOD: amrap 12 min
100m run
10 x TTB
100m run
10 x push ups

Session 1568
Strength
Deadlift - work to 3rm then 2 x 2 @ 95% of above weight

WOD: for time
8 x devil press (22.5/15)
5 x squat clean (60/40)

8 x devil press
4 x squat clean (70/45)

8 x devil press
3 x squat clean (80/55)

8 x devil press
2 x squat clean (90/60)

8 x devil press
1 x squat clean (100/65)

Session 1569

Partner amrap 40 min
400m kB carry (24/16)
100 x wallball
400m kB carry
100 x wallball sit ups
400m carry
Amrap 1 for 1 burpees in remainder

Session 1570

15/12/9
Push jerk (50/35)
Bar facing burpee

Rest

15/12/9
Box jump
Bar facing burpee

Rest

15/12/9
Db hang power clean
Bar facing burpee

Session 1571
Strength/skill:
Weighted negative pull ups - accumulate 10-15 reps

WOD: 3 rounds for time
15 x pull up
20 x kB swing (24/16)
800m run

Session 1572
Strength/skill:
Hang squat clean/squat clean - work to heavy

WOD: 2 min window
25 x wallball
30 x double unders
Max hang squat clean (60/40)

Rest 2 min
Repeat x 5 rounds
*if fail to get to cleans drop reps x 5

Session 1573
Strength/skill:
Hang power snatch/ power snatch - work to heavy

WOD: 3 rounds for time
30 x KTE
10 x Turkish get up (15/10)

Session 1574

Strength/skill:
Deadlift - 2 x 3 @last weeks top weight

WOD: amrap 18 min
8 x Db snatch (22.5/15)
8 x burpee
1 x bear complex (40/30)

*increase bear complex x 1 each round

Session 1575

40 min strongman

WOD: amrap 8 min
1 x left arm DB thruster
1 x right arm thruster
5 x pull up
*increase thrusters x 1 rep each round

Session 1576

5 Rounds for time
26 x walking lunges
5 x bar muscle ups

Rest

4 rounds for time
12 x front squat (60/40) *no rack
50 x double unders

Session 1577

Strength/skill:
Front - squat 1 & 1/4's
3 x 3

WOD: for time
200m O/H plate carry (20/15)
15 x hang power clean (40/30)
200m FARMER carry (22.5/15)
10 x hang power clean (60/40)
200m FARMER carry
5 x hang power clean (80/55)
200m O/H plate carry

Session 1578

Strength/skill:
Bench press 5 x 5

WOD: 2 rounds for time
15 x renegade row (22.5/15)
20 x left arm Db push jerk
15 x renegade row
20 x right arm Db push jerk

Session 1579
Deadlift- 5x5

WOD: amrap 12 min
200m run
14 x box jump
200m run
7 x burpee pull up

Session 1580

Ascending Partner amrap 40 min
10 cal bike or row
30 x kB swing

20 cal
30 x kB swing

30 cal
30 x kB swing

40 cal
20 x kB CLEAN & JERK

50 cal
20 x kB clean and jerk

60 cal
20 x kB clean and jerk

70 cal
10 x synchro KB SNATCH

80 cal
10 x synchro snatch

90 cal
10 x synchro snatch

Session 1581

3 rounds for time
10 x burpee over Db's
15 x Db clean and jerk (22.5/15)

Rest

5 rounds for time
5 x hang power clean (70/50)
15 x wallball

Session 1582

Strength/skill:
Front squat 5 x 2
*3 second pause at bottom position

WOD: amrap 8 min
12 x single arm overhead DB lunge (22.5/15)
18 x DB snatch

Rest

1 min max cals assault bike

Session 1583

Strength/skill:
Ring dips 5 x max effort
Or
5 x 10 assisted

WOD: 3 rounds for time
20 x pull up
30 x plate snatch (20/15)
400 m run

Session 1584

Strength/skill:
Hang squat clean - 3/3/2/2/1/1

WOD: 1 min window
25 air squat
Amrap c+j (60/40)
Rest 1 min
Repeat x 8

Session 1585

40 min strongman

Amrap 8 min
10 x renegade row
5 x Db hang squat clean

Session 1586

15/12/9
Cluster (60/40)
L-sit pull up

Rest

Amrap 12
2 x muscle up
4 x jumping lunge (each leg)
8 x kB swing (24/16)

Session 1587

Strength/skill:
Push press - 5 x 5

WOD: amrap 12 min
8 x hspu
16 x wallball
24 x double unders

Session 1588
Strength/skill:
Turkish get up - over 10-12 reps work to a heavy.

WOD: 10-1
TTB
Db box step overs (22,5/15)
*2 x clean and jerk after each round (60/40)

Session 1589

Strength/skill:
Overhead squat - 5 x 3
*3 sec pause at bottom

WOD: 3 min window
15 x pull up
15 x push up
15 x squat

Max effort devils press

Rest 90 sec
Repeat x 5

Session 1590

Strength/skill
Deadlift 5 x 5

WOD: amrap 7 min
6 x Db snatch
2 x burpee box jump
*increase burpee box x each round

Session 1591

Partner Amrap 40 min
5 x synchro med ball clean
5 x synchro push ups
10 x cal bike/row (half each)

10 x synchro ball clean
10 x synchro push ups
20 x cal bike/row (half each)

15 x synchro ball clean
15 x synchro push ups
30 x cal bike/row

20 x synchro ball clean
20 x synchro push ups
40 x cal bike/row

Etc... continue adding 5 reps to cleans and push ups. Cals = combined reps of bike and push ups

Session 1592

5/4/3/2/1
Rope climb
400 m run after each climb

Rest

8 min amrap
12 x Db thruster (22.5/15)
12 x kB sumo high pull (24/16)

Session 1593

Strength/skill:
Weighted pull up - 5 x 5

WOD- for time
100 x double under
4 x clean and jerk (70/45)
50 x sit up
3 x clean and jerk
75 x box jump
2 x clean and jerk
50 x sit up
1 x clean and jerk
100 x double under

Session 1594
Strength/skill:

Back squat 3 x 10

WOD: 3 rounds for time
30 x wallball
20 x ttb
10 x front rack lunge (40/30)

Session 1595

Strength/skill:
Power clean 5 x 3
*reset each rep, light and snappy 70% 'Ish

WOD: Ascending ladder 15 min
Hang power clean x 2 (60/40)
Renegade row x 2
*increase x 2 reps

Session 1596

Strength/skill:
Strict press 4 x 7

WOD: 2 rounds for time
30 x burpee
25 x kB swing (24/16)
20 x thruster (40/30)
15 x pull up

Session 1597

Strength/skill:
3rft
21 x wallball
15 x hspu

9 x ttb

Rest

21/15/9
Hang power snatch (40/30)
Chest to bar pull up

Session 1597

Strength/skill:
Ring dips - 5 x max effort

WOD: 2 min window
30 x double unders
10 x burpee
Max single arm Db hang clean and jerk
Rest 1 min repeat
Continue untill 60 Db clean and jerks complete.
*capped at 7 rounds

Session 1598
Strength/skill:
Push press 1rm

WOD: Amrap 7 min
20 x push up
20 x KB sumo high pull (24/16)

Rest 3 min

Amrap - 7 min
10 x pull up
20 x sit up

Session 1599
Strength/skill:

Front squat 1rm

WOD: 3 rounds for time
1a2 x cluster (60/40)
15 x ttb
18 x Db snatch (22.5/15)

Session 1600

40 min strongman

WOD: amrap 10 min
7 x pull up
10 x push
7 x wallball

Session 1601

3 rounds for time
400m run
15 x thruster (40/30)
3 x rope climb

Rest

For time
25 x pull up
25 x burpee
50 x burpee pull up

Session 1602
Strength/skill:
Dynamic effort box squat
10 x 3 @ 65% EMOM

WOD: 18 min ascending ladder
2 x Db box step overs (22.5/15)
2 x Db burpee deadlift
2 x box jump
*increase x 2

Session 1603
Strength/skill:
Bench press 3rm

WOD: for time
75 x sit up
50 x Db snatch (22.5/15)
10 x DB squat clean (AHAP)
50 x Db snatch
75 x sit up

Session 1604

Strength/skill:
Power clean 3rm

WOD: for time
400m run
9 x hang clean and jerk (60/40)
400m run
12 x hang clean and jerk
400m run
15 x hang clean and jerk
400m run

Session 1605

Strength/skill:
Front squat 3rm
Back squat - 20 reps @ 80% - 10kg

WOD: amrap 12
120 x wallball
30 x muscle up
*scaled to burpee pull-ups

Session 1606

40 min AMRAP

100 cal bike/row
100 x single arm thrusters
50 cal bike/row
50 x Db snatch
25 cal bike/row
25 x synchro sit ups

Session 1607

2 rounds for time
80 x double unders
40 x air squat
20 x deadlift (80/60)

Rest

9/15/21
Hang power clean (60/40)
Box jump

Session 1608

Strength/skill:
Dynamic effort box squat
12 x 2 @ 55%

WOD: 3 min window
400m run
Max effort burpee pull up
Rest 1 min
Repeat x 5 rounds

Session 1609
Strength/skill:
Weighted ring dips - 5 x 5

WOD: 10 rounds for time
20 x kb swing (24/16)
15 x sit up
2 x Turkish get up (15/10)

Session 1610

Strength/skill:
Hang power snatch work to heavy 3

WOD: 12 min amrap
1 x power snatch (50/35) *increase x1
10 x push up
25 x double under

Session 1611

Front squat- 5rm
Back squat 20 reps 80% - 15kg

WOD: 3 rounds for time
20 x right arm oh Db lunge (22.5/15)
10 x Ttb
20 x left arm oh Db lunge
10 x pull up

Session 1612
40 min strongman

10 min ascending ladder
2 x air squat
2 x burpee
2 x Db snatch

*increase reps x 2 each round

Session 1613

5 rounds for time
9 x thruster (50/35)

1 x legless rope climb

Rest

7 rounds for time
7 x hspu
6 x pull up
5 x hang power snatch (50/35)

Session 1614
Strength/skill:
Dynamic effort box squat
10 x 2 @ 70% Emom

WOD: for time
50 x box jump
1 x cluster (70/47.5)
50 x push up
2 x cluster
50 x wallball
3 x cluster
50 x KTE
4 x cluster

Session 1615

Strength/skill:
Power clean 5 x 1

WOD: amrap 12 min

8 x Sumo high pull (60/40)
32 x sit ups
100m overhead plate carry (20/15)

Session 1616

Strength/skill:
Push press -work to 2rm
Then 2 extra sets of 2 @ 90%

WOD: every 3 min start a new round x 6 rounds

10 x burpee
12 x double DB hang snatch (22.5/15)
10 x pull up (*incease x 1 each round)

Session 1617
Strength/skill:
Front squat heavy 2
Back squat x 20 reps @ 80% -20kg

WOD: 10 - 1 reps of
DB power clean (22.5/15)
DB lunge (in rack position)
*reps per leg, e.g 10 reps EACH leg

Session 1618

40 min partner amrap
Partner A - 400m run
Partner B - chip away at list
Swap upon partner A return

50 x Man makers
50 x sit ups
50 cal bike / row
50 x devils press
50 x sit ups
50 cal bike / row

Session 1619

Amrap 12
1 x round of Cindy
1 x round of DT

*cindy - 5 x pull up, 10 x push up, 15 x squat
*DT - 12 x deadlift, 9 x hang power clean, 6 x push jerk (70/45)

Rest

For time

100 x burpee
Emom 5 x ttb

Session 1620

Strength/skill:
Dynamic effort box squat
10 x 2 @60%

WOD: 2 min window
2 x bear complex (40/30)
Max effort box jump

Rest 2 min
Repeat x 6 rounds
*increase complex x 1 each round
*if can't complete reps of complex in time frame go back a rep

Session 1621

Strength/skill:
Snatch grip deadlift- 5 x 5

WOD: amrap 10 min
80 x double unders
20 x DB snatch (22.5/15)
10 x burpee over Db

Session 1622

Strength/skill:
Pull up 4 x max effort
Or
Accumulate 15-20 negative reps

WOD: 3 rounds for time
12 x renegade row (22.5/15)
800m run

Session 1623
Strength/skill:
Front squat
heavyish 3rep

Back squat 20 reps. 5kg heavier than last week. (Should be 80% - 25kg)

WOD: for time
200 walking lunges (*can jump)
Emom 1 x cluster (60/40)

Session 1624

40 min strongman

WOD: amrap 10 min
20 x kB swing
20 x sit ups
20 x jumping lunges

Session 1625

9 rounds for time
1 x clean and jerk (75%)
3 x l-sit pull up
5 x ring dips
7 x DB lunge (22.5/15)

Rest

For time
50 x burpee box overs

Session 1626
Strength/skill:
Dynamic effort Box squat (just below parallel) - 10 x 2 @ 50% EMOM

WOD: 90 sec window
3 x sumo high pull (40/30)
3 x thruster
3 x hang power clean

Max effort double unders

90 sec rest
Repeat x 7 rounds
*increase x 1 rep every round
*if you get to a round you can't complete all barbell movements go back a rep

Session 1627

Strength/skill:
Bench press - 5 x 3 (pause on chest each rep)

WOD: amrap 12 min
10 x Db box step over (22.5/15)
15 x box jump
E2mom - 3 x clean and jerk (60/40)

Session 1628
Strength/skill:
Find heavy complex-
Power snatch/overhead squat/hang squat snatch

WOD: 3 rounds for time
24 x Db snatch (22.5/15)
16 x burpee
8 x ttb

Session 1629

Strength/skill:
Front squat - heavyish 5
Back squat 1 x 20 (starting weight is 80% of 1rm then - 30kg)
*(will be adding 5kg each week)

WOD - 20.5

Session 1630

In pairs
40 min clock
200 cal row/bike

Into amrap in remainder
60 x burpee over partner
60 x synchro KB clean & jerk

30 x burpee over partner
30 x plate snatch

100 x synchro devils press

Session 1631

10-1
Pull up strict
Strict press (35/25)
Box jump

Rest

5 rounds for time
15 x power clean (40/30)
15 x wallball

Session 1632
Strength/skill:
Hang power clean 5 x 2

WOD: 12 min amrap
12 x overhead lunge (40/30)
15 x TTB
27 x double unders

Session 1633

Strength/skill:
Strict press 3x3
Push press 3x3

WOD: for time
15 x rounds of "Cindy"

5 x pull
10 x push up
15 x squat

Emom - 6 x Db snatch

Session 1634

40 min strongman

WOD: amrap 10 min
12 x medball clean
12 x push up
12 x ring row

Session 1635

15/12/9/6/3
DB burpee
DB thruster

Rest

21/15/9
DB snatch
Pull up

If time allows
Secret Bonus WOD

Session 1636

Strength/skill:
Clean and jerk - work to 2rm

WOD: amrap 9 min
2 x Hang power clean (60/40)
10 x box jump
*increase clean x2 each round

Session 1637
Strength/skill:
Pendlay row 5 x 5

WOD: for time
75 x wallball
150 x sit up
75 x wallball

Session 1638
Strength/skill:
Overhead lunge - 3 x 10 (5 each leg)

WOD: 8 rounds for time
8 x burpee
100m run
8 x pull up
100m run

Session 1639
Strength/skill:
Push press 5 x 5

WOD : open WOD 20.3
21/15/9
Deadlift (102/70)
Hspu
Into
21/15/9
Deadlift
Handstand walk 50ft

9min cap

Session 1640

5 rounds for time
50 double double
15 x push press (35/25
10 x toes to bar

Rest

For time
50 x Db burpee deadlift (22.5/15)

Session 1641

Strength/skill:
Deficit deadlift 3 x 3 AHAP

WOD: 3 min window
10 x pull up
10 x burpee
10 x kB swing (24/16)
Max effort jumping lunge holding medball

Rest 60 sec
Repeat x 5 rounds

*if you have longer than 30 sec of lunges
Increase reps x 2

Session 1642
Weighted Ring dip 5 x 5

WOD: amrap 20min
30 x sit up
15 x box jump
2 x single arm DB cluster (22.5/15)
*incease cluster x2 each round

Session 1643
Strength/skill:
Squat snatch - work up to heavy

WOD: 3 rounds for time
10 x hang clean and jerk (50/35)
800m run

18/10/19
3 rounds for time
20 x thruster (40/30)
15 x ttb
10 x hang power clean

Rest

Amrap 14 min
50 x double under
12 x sumo high pull (40/30)
2 x rope climb

Session 1644
Strength/skill:
Overhead squat 5 x 3

WOD: for time
50 x devils press (22.5/15)
Emom - 5 x box jump

Session 1645

Strength/skill:
Pendlay row - 5x5

WOD: 5 rounds for time
12 x pull up
18 x wallball

Session 1646

Strength/skill:
Db push jerk 5 x 5 (single arm)

WOD: amrap 20 min
12 x hspu
24 x kB swing (24/16)
36 x o/h kB lunge

Session 1647

For time as a 2 person team

400 x double unders
200 x sit ups
100 x squat clean
50 x rope climb

Session 1648

Strength/skill:
Push jerk 5 x 3

WOD: amrap 12 min
Deadlift x 5 (100/70)
Kb clean and jerk x 10 (24/16)
Push up x 15

Session 1649

Strength/skill:
Front rack lunge- 4 x 10m

WOD: 5 rounds for time
20 x wallball
10 x box jump
20 x sit up

Session 1650
Strength/skill:
1rm bench press

WOD: 10 rounds for time
5 x Db hang power clean (22.5/15)
5 x burpee over Db
5 x pull up

Session 1651
Strength/skill:
Hang squat clean - 2rm

WOD: amrap 14 min

Clean and jerk x 1
Toes to bar x 10
Double under x 50

*increase clean and jerk x 1

Session 1652

4 rounds for time
25 x thruster (20/15)
5 x ring muscle up

Rest

4 rounds for time
24 x front rack lunge (30/25)
18 x hang power clean
12 x push jerk

Session 1653

Strength/skill:
Sumo high pull - 5 x 5

WOD: amrap - 9 min
1 x Hang power snatch (40/30)
5 x bar over burpee

*increase snatch x 1 each round

Session 1654
Strength/skill:
Weighted pull up 5 x 5

WOD: 30/20/10
Renegade row (22.5/15) *no push up
Plate snatch (20/15)
100m over head plate carry after each round

Session 1655

Strength/skill:
1 rm strict press

WOD: amrap 5 min
3 x power clean (60/40)
6 x push up
9 x air squat
Rest 1 min
Repeat x 4 rounds

Session 1656
Strength/skill:
Squat clean 3rm

WOD:

WOD: for time
50 x ttb
5 x dball squat clean (ahap)
50 x kB swing
4 x dball squat clean
50 x sit ups
3 x dball squat clean
50 x hollow rocks
2 x dball squat clean
50 x v -ups

1 x dball squat clean

Session 1657

Strength/skill:
Deadlift 1rm

WOD: 2 min window
12 x HR push up
12 x DB Snatch (22.5/15)
Max effort wallball

1 min rest
Repeat x 5 rounds

Session 1658

Strength/skill:
L - sit: accumulate 3 min
Ring dip support: accumulate 3 min

WOD: amrap 25 min
400m run
12 x Turkish ups (15/10)
24 x single Db hang clean and jerk (same Db, alternating)

Session 1659

Strength/skill:
Hang power snatch 2rm

WOD: 5 rounds for time
15 x kb swing (24/16)
10 x pull up
5 x ttb
50 x double unders

Printed in the USA
CPSIA information can be obtained
at www.ICGtesting.com
LVHW061944310823
756864LV00011BA/341